The Comfort
of Home®
for Chronic Heart Failure

A Guide for Caregivers

The Comfort of Home® Caregiver book series is written for family and paraprofessional home caregivers who face the responsibilities of caring for aging friends, family, or clients. The disease-specific editions, often in collaboration with organizations supporting those conditions, address caregivers assisting people with those diseases.

Other Caregiver Resources from CareTrust Publications:

La comodidad del hogar® (Spanish Edition)
The Comfort of Home®: A Complete Guide for Caregivers
The Comfort of Home® for Chronic Lung Disease
The Comfort of Home® for Chronic Liver Disease
The Comfort of Home® for Alzheimer's Disease
The Comfort of Home® Multiple Sclerosis Edition
The Comfort of Home® for Parkinson Disease
The Comfort of Home® for Stroke
The Comfort of Home® Caregiving Journal
Caring in The Comfort of Home® UK Edition
The Comfort of Home® Caregivers—Let's Take Care of You! Meditation CD

Newsletters:

The Comfort of Home® Caregiver Assistance News
The Comfort of Home® Grand-Parenting News
The Comfort of Home® Caregivers—Let's Take Care of You!

Visit *www.comfortofhome.com* for forthcoming editions and other caregiver resources.

The Comfort of Home®

for Chronic Heart Failure

A Guide for Caregivers

Maria M. Meyer *and* Paula Derr, RN

with

Kay Kendall, MSW, LISW *and* Jennifer Reese, RN, BSN

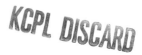
CareTrust Publications LLC
"Caring for you... caring for others."
Portland, Oregon

The Comfort of Home® for Chronic Heart Failure: A Guide for Caregivers

Published by: CareTrust Publications LLC
P.O. Box 10283
Portland, Oregon 97296-0283
(800) 565-1533
Fax (503) 221-7019
www.comfortofhome.com

Publisher's Cataloging-in-Publication
(Provided by Quality Books, Inc.)

Meyer, Maria M., 1948-
　　The comfort of home for chronic heart failure:
　a guide for caregivers / Maria M. Meyer and Paula Derr
　with Kay Kendall and Jennifer Reese
　　　　p. cm.
　　　　Includes index.
　　　　ISBN-13: 978-0-9787903-3-2
　　　　ISBN-10: 0-9787903-3-2

　　1. Home care services--Handbooks, manuals, etc.
　2. Caregivers--Handbooks, manuals, etc.　3. Heart failure.
　4. Chronic diseases. I. Derr, Paula.　II. Title.

RA645.3.M4937 2008　　　　　　　649.8
　　　　　　　　　　　　　　　QBI08-860

Cover Art and Text Illustration: Stacey L. Tandberg
Interior Design: Frank Loose
Cover Design: David Kessler
Editor: Jon Caswell
Page Layout: Lapiz

Distributed to the Trade by Publishers Group West.
Printed in the United States of America.

08 09 10 11 12/10 9 8 7 6 5 4 3 2 1

About the Authors

Maria M. Meyer has been a long-time advocate of social causes, beginning with her work as co-founder of the Society for Abused Children of the Children's Home Society of Florida and founding executive director of the Children's Foundation of Greater Miami. When her father-in-law suffered a stroke in 1993, Maria became aware of the need for better information about how to care for an aging parent, a responsibility shared by millions of Americans. That experience led Maria to found CareTrust Publications and to co-author the award-winning guide, *The Comfort of Home®: An Illustrated Step-by-Step Guide for Caregivers*—now in its third edition. This book earned the Benjamin Franklin Award in the health category, as well as *Finalist* in ForeWord Magazine's 2007 Book of the Year Award. She is a keynote speaker and workshop leader on caregiver topics to health care professionals and community groups, as well as a Caregiver Community Action Network volunteer for the National Family Caregiver Association.

Paula Derr, RN, BSN, CEN, CCRN, has been employed by the Sisters of Providence Health System for over 30 years. She has broad experience in many different clinical settings and for many years served as clinical educator for three emergency departments in the Portland metropolitan area. She was a founder of InforMed, which publishes emergency medical services field guides for emergency medical technicians (EMTs), paramedics, firefighters, physicians, and nurses, and has co-authored numerous health care articles. For Paula, home care is a family tradition of long standing. For many years, Paula cared for her mother and grandmother in her home while raising two daughters and maintaining her career in nursing and health care management. Her personal and professional experience adds depth to many chapters of this book. Paula is active in several prominent professional organizations and has held both local and national board positions. Paula is a native Oregonian and lives with her husband in Portland.

Kay Kendall, MSW, LISW, ACSW, has been a licensed, clinical social worker for over 30 years. For the first 15 years of her career, she provided individual, marital, and family counseling in a variety of settings. In 1989, after moving to Cleveland with her husband and two sons, Kay began working at the Cleveland Clinic with cardiac patients and their families. As a member of the Cleveland Clinic Heart Failure/Heart Transplant Team, Kay provides ongoing counseling and support to both patients and their families. Through daily contact, she counsels patients and their families as they adjust and adapt to managing a chronic medical condition. Through the years she has spent in the hospital setting, Kay has come to recognize the significance of the caregiver in the treatment process, and the role of the patient and their family in disease management, and outcome. Kay has published articles on the quality of life of patients with heart failure, the stages and process through which patients adjust to illness, and ways to improve compliance with medical recommendations. She has also presented at national and international conferences. Kay served for five years as the President of the Society for Transplant Social Workers, and she remains active on their executive board.

Jennifer Reese, RN, BSN, has been employed by the Cleveland Clinic for the past 10 years. After graduating from nursing school, her focus has been in cardiac care. She started her career in the cardiac intensive care units, before joining the Heart Failure/Heart Transplant Team. As a member of this team she provides ongoing care and education for both the heart failure and heart transplant patients and their families. She has been involved in several task forces and committees at the Cleveland Clinic to help improve the quality of care that both patients and their families receive. Jennifer has presented at several national conferences and provides educational lectures to other community hospitals and facilities on the care of both the heart failure and heart transplant patient. She is active in several professional organizations both locally and internationally and volunteers for several local charitable organizations. Jennifer continues on in her educational career by pursuing her Adult Nurse Practitioner degree at a local university. She is a native Ohioan and lives with her daughter.

Our Mission

CareTrust Publications is committed to providing high-quality,
user-friendly information to those who face an illness or the
responsibilities of caring for friends, family, or clients.

Dedication

*To our heart failure patients whom we have worked
with, cared for and learned from.*
—Kay Kendall and Jennifer Reese

Dear Caregiver,

When a family member is diagnosed with chronic heart failure, you, the caregiver, will have to know and understand how the disease needs to be treated and what level of care is required.

The Comfort of Home® for Chronic Heart Failure: A Guide for Caregivers is a basic, complete guide that will answer your questions about caregiving. Covering current best practices for home care, it offers practical tips for everyday problems as well as more complicated and stressful situations, such as learning about the progression of the disease and end-of-life decisions.

The *Guide* is divided into three parts:

Part One, Getting Ready, describes the types of chronic heart failure and how the disease affects the person for whom you care. You will learn about the basic function of the heart, the symptoms of heart failure and the typical path that this disease follows.

Part Two, Day-by-Day tells you how to develop a daily schedule, and understand the challenges of living with chronic heart failure and its special care needs, such as taking medications as prescribed, following dietary recommendations, and working with the heart failure medical team.

Part Three, Additional Resources, provides a glossary of common medical terms to help you understand the language that many health care professionals use to talk about chronic heart failure. It also includes a list of references for further reading and information about organizations and publications for caregivers.

Armed with knowledge, you will feel confident that you can provide good care. With this *Guide* in hand, you will understand what help is needed and learn where to find it or how to provide it yourself.

Warm regards,

Maria, Paula, Kay & Jennifer

Maria, Paula, Kay and Jennifer

Acknowledgments

The information in this *Guide* is based on research and consultation with experts in the fields of nursing, medicine, and design. The authors thank the innumerable professionals and caregivers who have assisted in the development of this book.

This volume would not have been possible without the support of our colleagues and our families.

Special thanks go to the following people who shared their expertise in caring for those with chronic heart failure. They kindly offered information and support:

Rebecca Armagno, RN
Case Manager/Home Care Nurse

Diane L. Nowak RD, LD
Registered Dietitian
The Cleveland Clinic

David O. Taylor, MD, FACC
Professor of Medicine
Director, Heart Failure Special Care Unit
Director, HF and Cardiac Transplant Fellowship Program
The Cleveland Clinic

Megan Goheen, RN
Hospice of the Western Reserve
Cleveland, Ohio

Sheila Delson
Financial Coordinator
Transplant Center
The Cleveland Clinic

Some sections of this volume are adapted from other editions in the *Comfort of Home®* series. We extend our gratitude to those authors and organizations whose contributions have enhanced this book.

To Our Readers

We believe *The Comfort of Home® for Chronic Heart Failure: A Guide for Caregivers* reflects currently accepted practice in the areas it covers. However, the authors and publisher assume no liability with respect to the accuracy, completeness, or application of information presented here.

The Comfort of Home® for Chronic Heart Failure is not meant to replace medical care but to add to the medical advice and services you receive from health care professionals. You should seek professional medical advice from a health care provider. This book is only a guide; follow your common sense and good judgment.

Neither the authors nor the publisher are engaged in rendering legal, accounting, or other professional advice. Seek the services of a competent professional if legal, architectural, or other expert assistance is required. The *Guide* does not represent Americans with Disabilities Act compliance.

Every effort has been made at the time of publication to provide accurate names, addresses, and phone numbers in the resource sections at the ends of chapters. The resources listed are those that benefit readers nationally. For this reason, we have not included many local groups that offer valuable assistance. Failure to include an organization does not mean that it does not provide a valuable service. On the other hand, inclusion does not imply an endorsement. The authors and publisher do not warrant or guarantee any of the products described in this book and did not perform any independent analysis of the products described.

Throughout the book, we use "he" and "she" interchangeably when referring to the caregiver and the person being cared for.

ATTENTION NONPROFIT ORGANIZATIONS, CORPORATIONS, AND PROFESSIONAL ORGANIZATIONS: *The Comfort of Home® for Chronic Heart Failure* is available at special quantity discounts for bulk purchases for gifts, fundraising, or educational training purposes. Special books, book excerpts, or booklets can also be created to fit specific needs. For details, write to CareTrust Publications LLC, P.O. Box 10283, Portland, Oregon 97296-0283, or call 1-800-565-1533.

CONTENTS AT A GLANCE

Praise for *The Comfort of Home*® Caregiver Guides

"This is an invaluable addition to bibliographies for the home caregiver. Hospital libraries will want to have a copy on hand for physicians, nurses, social workers, chaplains, and any staff dealing with MS patients and their caregivers. Highly recommended for all public libraries and consumer health collections."
—*Library Journal*

"A well-organized format with critical information and resources at your fingertips . . . educates the reader about the many issues that stand before people living with chronic conditions and provides answers and avenues for getting the best care possible."
—MSWorld, Inc. www.msworld.org

"A masterful job of presenting the multiple aspects of caregiving in a format that is both comprehensive and reader-friendly . . . important focus on physical aspects of giving care."
—Parkinson Report

"Almost any issue or question or need for resolution is most likely spoken of somewhere within the pages of this guide."
—*American Journal of Alzheimer's Disease*

"Physicians, family practitioners and geriatricians, and hospital social workers should be familiar with the book and recommend it to families of the elderly."
—Reviewers Choice, Home Care University

"An excellent guide on caregiving in the home. Home health professionals will find it to be a useful tool in teaching family caregivers."
—Five Star Rating, *Doody's Health Sciences Review Journal*

"Overall a beautifully designed book with very useful, practical information for caregivers."
—Judges from the Benjamin Franklin Awards

"Noteable here are the specifics. Where others focus on psychology alone, this gets down to the nitty gritty."
—*The Midwest Book Review*

"We use *The Comfort of Home*® for the foundational text in our 40-hour Caregiver training. I believe it is the best on the market."
—Linda Young, Project Manager, College of the Desert

Part One: Getting Ready

What is Heart Failure?

What Is Heart Failure?

*H*eart failure is a chronic medical condition that affects over 5 million people in the United States. It is a manageable disease, but is not curable. Heart failure progresses differently in each person depending on age, additional medical problems, and how a person cares for themselves. The symptoms of heart failure are:

- *Shortness of breath (also called dyspnea [dis-PEE-nia])*

- *Persistent coughing or wheezing*

- *Buildup of excess fluid in body tissues (edema [e-DE-ma])*

- *Tiredness, fatigue*

- *Lack of appetite, nausea*

- *Confusion, impaired thinking*

- *Increased heart rate*

> **NOTE** There are 500,000 new cases diagnosed each year. Heart failure is most common in people 65 years and older. Ten percent of those who reach the age of 75 are diagnosed with heart failure.

The progression of heart failure varies with individuals. Age and the presence of other medical problems affect how the disease advances. Many individuals function independently for a long time and gradually need more assistance from a caregiver. But conditions can change quickly, and the person in your care may eventually require more help. As heart failure advances, that person may need total care.

As medical conditions change, the heart failure patient's mood may also change. Some become discouraged when they first learn of their diagnosis. Others become depressed and anxious as their daily activities become more and more limited. We discuss mood changes and what can help in **Chapter 14, Special Challenges.**

It is very important that you know from the beginning that you have to find ways to take care of yourself. This self-care is not a luxury, it is a necessity, and you have to make it happen. Maybe you fit a walk in while the person in your care is napping, or do 10 minutes of yoga after he has gone to bed, or you might read a book before he wakes up. Whatever you do, do something every day, even if it's just a little bit.

> **NOTE** ▸ Here's why *every day* is so important: Stress builds, grows, and accumulates. You can't take stress away from caregiving, but you can reduce it. To do so you have to take care of yourself in some way each day. Think of this time—walking, reading, bathing, meditating—whatever you choose, as a break in your day when you can think about your needs, even if just for a few minutes. Decide now that you will do this for yourself. It will make a big difference in how you feel.

What Is Heart Failure?

Heart failure means that the heart is pumping less volume than normal. It does not mean that the heart has stopped working, just that it is weaker than normal. Heart failure usually develops over many years, therefore, people often don't even know they have it until symptoms such as shortness of breath or swelling appear years after changes began.

With heart failure, the pressure in the heart increases because the blood moves through the heart and body at a slower rate. As the heart pumps less and less efficiently, the body's need for oxygen and nutrients are not met. The chambers of the heart respond to this inefficiency by stretching to hold more blood to pump through the body. This weakens the muscle walls and causes them to not pump as strongly. This results in fatigue, fluid retention, and shortness of breath, making everyday activities such as bathing and dressing or climbing a flight of stairs difficult. If fluid builds up in the body (for example, the arms, legs, feet, lungs, or other organs), the body becomes swollen or congested, which is why this disease is often referred to as **congestive heart failure**. The severity of the heart failure determines the impact on a person's life. Mild heart failure may have little effect, yet severe heart failure can interfere with simple activities, such as bathing and dressing, and can even prove fatal.

Heart failure is a condition that has no cure, but with the right treatment, consisting of medications and lifestyle changes, people can live full and pleasurable lives. It also helps to have a caregiver who understands the condition.

How the Normal Heart Works

To fully understand heart failure, let's first take a look at how the normal heart works. To pump blood effectively through the body, a healthy, normal heart beats between 60 and 80 times per minute.

Imagine the normal heart as the body's engine; it needs enough oil, gas, and transmission fluid to run properly. Without these fluids, the engine will not function properly, either stalling or shutting down completely. Performing proper maintenance keeps your engine running smoothly, as taking care of yourself keeps your normal heart healthy. Sometimes, despite proper maintenance, problems still develop.

The heart has two sides that are separated by a wall of muscle called the *septum*. Blood returning from the body enters the upper right chamber of the heart, called the *right atrium*. From there it goes into the lower chamber, called the *right ventricle* by way of the tricuspid valve. From there the blood is pushed through the pulmonary artery into the lungs, where oxygen is added. This oxygen-rich blood then enters the upper left chamber of the heart (called the *left atrium*) and then goes to the lower chamber (called the *left ventricle*). At that point, it moves, via the mitral valve, into blood vessels (arteries), which carry the blood to the body.

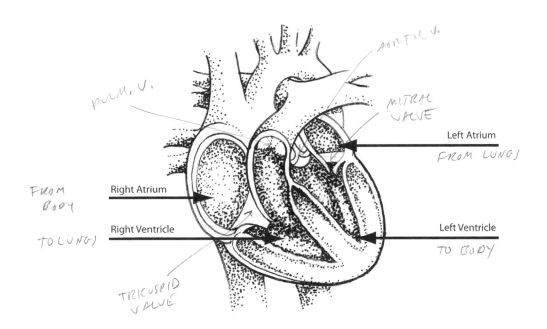

In addition to four chambers, the heart also has four valves, which open and shut like doors. When open, they allow blood to move to the next chamber; and when shut they keep blood from going backwards. These four valves are:

- The tricuspid valve, in the right side of the heart, between the upper chamber (right atrium) and lower chamber (right ventricle).

- The pulmonary valve, also in the right side of the heart, between the lower chamber (right ventricle) and the vessel that carries blood to the lungs (pulmonary artery).

- The mitral valve, between the left atrium and left ventricle.

- The aortic valve, also in the left side of the heart, between the left ventricle and the aorta, which is the large artery that carries blood to the body.

Types of Heart Failure

As a caregiver, you may accompany the person in your care to some or all of her doctor appointments. At these visits, you may hear the physician refer to her heart failure as "left-sided" or "right-sided" heart failure, or as "systolic" or "diastolic" heart failure. Let's look in more detail at these different types.

Left-sided heart failure

Left-sided heart failure (also known as *left ventricular heart failure*) involves the lower chamber (left ventricle) of the heart. The left ventricle is the part of the heart that pumps the oxygen-rich blood to the rest of the body. Because of this, the left ventricle has a lot of pumping power, thus making it slightly larger than the other three chambers of the heart. If the left ventricle doesn't contract with enough force, it is not able to pump enough of this oxygen-rich blood to the rest of the body. (This is called "systolic heart failure.") If the left ventricle is able to contract normally but is stiff and can't relax enough, then blood cannot enter the heart. (This is called "diastolic heart failure.") In either case, the left ventricle responds by stretching to hold more blood to pump through the body, which weakens the muscle wall, causing it to pump less strongly.

LV STRETCHES → WEAKER → PUMPS LESS STRONGLY

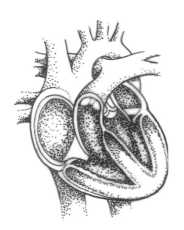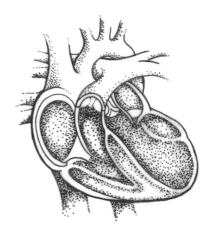

The two pictures above show the difference between a normal left ventricle (left) and left ventricle affected by heart failure (right).

Right-sided heart failure

Right-sided heart failure (also known as *right ventricular heart failure*) is usually a result of left ventricular failure. Because the right and left sides of the heart work together, when the left ventricle fails, this eventually increases the burden on the right ventricle, causing it to fail as well. If the right side of the heart does not deliver enough blood supply to the left side of the heart, then this blood backs up in the body's veins, causing swelling, usually in the legs and ankles. Right ventricular failure alone is very rare, but when it does happen, it is difficult to manage and patients are usually more symptomatic.

Causes of Heart Failure

All people lose some of their heart's pumping ability as they age, but with heart failure there is a more significant loss. Heart failure is caused by many conditions that damage the heart muscle over time, leading to the decrease in pumping power. The three major causes of heart failure are **coronary artery disease, high blood pressure,** and **diabetes.**

Coronary Artery Disease

Coronary artery disease (also known as *coronary atheroscle-rosis* or *ischemic heart disease*) is a disease of the arteries that supply blood and oxygen to the heart. This occurs when the normal lining of the arteries breaks down, causing the walls to thicken, and fatty deposits (called *plaque*) block the flow of blood. Because these arteries become severely narrowed by these fatty deposits, the heart can no longer react to increased activity. The extra strain placed on the heart may result in high blood pressure (hypertension), chest pain (angina), or even a heart attack.

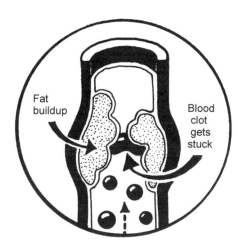

High Blood Pressure (Hypertension)

High blood pressure means that the pressure in the arteries is above normal range. Blood pressure is the pressure of the blood pushing against the walls of the arteries. Blood pressure is highest when the heart is pumping blood; this is called "systolic" pressure. Between beats, or when the heart is at rest, blood pressure falls; this is called "diastolic" pressure. High blood pressure, which is defined as a blood pressure reading of 140/90 mmHg or higher, usually has no symptoms. Sometimes people don't even know they have it until heart problems occur. Once it is diagnosed, it is very important to have it treated and monitored closely.

 Nearly 1 in 3 American adults has high blood pressure. Once high blood pressure develops, it usually lasts a lifetime. The good news is that it can be treated and controlled.

 In blood pressure measurement, the first (and larger) number represents systolic pressure, the pressure when the heart muscle is contracted. The second (and smaller) number is diastolic pressure, the pressure when the heart is between beats.

Diabetes Mellitus

Diabetes mellitus is defined as a fasting (tested on an empty stomach) blood sugar level of 126 mg/dL or more measured on two occasions. Diabetes is a disorder of metabolism, which is how our bodies use digested food for growth and energy. Most of the food we eat is broken down into glucose (sugar), which is the main source of fuel for the body.

After food is digested, this glucose passes into the bloodstream, where it is used by cells for growth and energy. For glucose to get into cells, insulin must be present. *Insulin* is a hormone produced by the pancreas (a gland behind the stomach). When we eat, the pancreas automatically produces the right amount of insulin to move glucose from the blood into the cells. However, in people with diabetes, the pancreas either produces little or no insulin, or the cells do not respond appropriately to the insulin that is produced. As a result, glucose builds up in the blood and then spills out of the body through urination. This results in the body losing its main source of fuel. Diabetes mellitus is associated with heart failure because it increases a person's risk of developing coronary artery disease. This condition, as discussed above, decreases the blood and oxygen supply to the heart.

NOTE Diabetes mellitus is Latin for "sweet urine."

Other Causes of Heart Failure

In addition to these three major causes, heart failure can also be caused by other heart diseases and conditions, including:

- **Cardiomyopathy**—damage to the heart muscle from something other than artery or blood flow problems

- **Arrhythmias**—abnormal heartbeats

- **Congenital heart defects**—a heart problem that a person is born with

- **Cancer treatments**—such as radiation or certain chemotherapy drugs

- **Alcohol or cocaine abuse**

- **Thyroid disorders**—having too much or too little thyroid hormone

- **Viral illness**

- **Diseases of the heart valves**

For more information on any of these diseases, you or the person in your care can go to your local library and ask a librarian to help you find more information. In addition, you can go to any one of the web sites listed in the resource section below for more information.

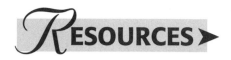

RESOURCES

Heart Failure Society of America, Inc.
Box 358
420 Delaware Street, SE
Minneapolis, MN 55455
Phone: (612) 626-3864
www.hfsa.org

American Heart Association
7272 Greenville Avenue
Dallas, TX 75231
Phone: (214) 373-6300 or
1-800-AHA-USA1
www.amhrt.org

National Heart, Lung and Blood Institute
National Institutes of Health
31 Center Drive, Bldg. 31, Room 5A52
Baltimore, MD 20892
Phone: (301) 496-4236
www.nhlbi.nih.gov

The Alliance for Aging Research
2021 K Street, NW
Suite 305
Washington, DC 20006
Phone: (202)293-2856
www.agingresearch.org

American College of Cardiology
www.acc.org/clinical/guidelines/failure

Heart Failure Risk Factors

Heart Failure Risk Factors

eart failure can happen to anyone, but it is more common in people over 65 years of age, among men and in African Americans. There are many traits and lifestyle habits (risk factors) that increase the chance of developing it. Some of these risk factors are controlled simply by changing lifestyle habits, while others are things that cannot be changed.

The person in your care likely has at least one risk factor. The best way to prevent heart failure is to reduce the risk factors that are controllable. Reducing risks generally results in improved quality of life. In addition, if you are a blood relative of the person you are caring for, you are at increased risk of heart failure yourself and should take steps to control your own risk factors. A doctor can help you change factors that result from lifestyle or the environment.

Controllable Risk Factors (things you can change)

Lifestyle changes may help reduce some of these risk factors, however, when lifestyle changes alone don't reduce these risk factors, ask a doctor for medical help.

Coronary Artery Disease (also known as coronary atherosclerosis)

Coronary artery disease is a disease of the arteries that supply blood and oxygen to the heart. It occurs when the normal lining of the arteries breaks down, causing the walls to thicken and fatty deposits (called plaque) block the flow of blood through these arteries. This is one of the three leading causes of heart failure, as well as a major contributor to high blood pressure.

High Blood Pressure

High blood pressure (140/90 mmHg or higher) is the second of the three leading causes of heart failure. It is referred to as "the silent killer" because it usually has no specific symptoms and no early warning signs. Both you and the person in your care should have your blood pressure checked regularly.

 NOTE Use a blood pressure cuff to monitor blood pressure at home. It's simple to use and gives a much better picture of the blood pressure of the person in your care than the readings taken on irregular trips to the doctor. Remember to keep a record of this to take to the doctor's office for review. See 📖 Chapter 10 *Setting up a Plan of Care* for an example of a self-care log.

Diabetes Mellitus

Again, this is defined as a fasting blood sugar level of 126 mg/dL or more measured on two occasions. This is the third of the three leading causes of heart failure. Even when diabetes is treated, having it still increases the risk of heart failure. If the person in your care has diabetes, work closely with her doctor to control it.

Smoking and Alcohol Abuse

Cigarette smoking is a major, preventable risk factor for heart disease. The nicotine and carbon monoxide in tobacco smoke reduce the oxygen in a person's blood, so smoking robs the heart of oxygen. Second-hand smoke is just as dangerous as first-hand smoke; therefore, ***if you or the person in your care smoke, get help to quit NOW!***

Alcohol can also damage the cells of the heart and make it harder for the heart to pump. Therefore, it is advised in people with heart failure to quit drinking alcohol.

> **NOTE** You may have read that drinking a glass or two of red wine a day is good for your heart, but this does not apply to the patient with heart failure. Check with the doctor if you have questions about alcohol consumption.

High Blood Cholesterol

A high level of total cholesterol is a major risk factor for coronary artery disease, which raises the risk of developing heart failure. Total cholesterol levels should be less than 200 mg/dL; LDL ("bad") levels (think of the L as *less desirable or lousy*) should be less than 100 mg/dL, while HDL (think of the H as *highly desirable or healthy*) should be between 40–60 mg/dL. *For more on cholesterol, see Chapter 15 on Diet, Nutrition, and Exercise.*

Physical Inactivity and Obesity

Inactivity and obesity both can increase the risk of high blood pressure, high blood cholesterol, diabetes, stroke and heart disease. Depending on his limitations, exercise may be difficult for the person in your care; nonetheless, it is very important. Therefore, find a way for him or her to be active. Ask your discharge planner about exercise options in your community.

Uncontrollable Risk Factors (things you *cannot* change)

Increasing Age

People of all ages, including children, can have heart failure. However, people 65 years and older have the highest proportion of heart failure, and the risk of heart failure increases with age. About 10 out of every 1,000 people older than 65 has heart failure and, since more people are living longer, heart failure is increasing.

Sex (gender)

In most age groups, more men than women are affected by heart failure. However, in terms of actual numbers, more women have heart failure because many more women live into their seventies and eighties, when heart failure is more common.

Heredity

Blood relatives of people who have cardiomyopathy are at increased risk for heart failure.

Race

African Americans are two to three times as likely as Caucasians to have heart failure. This may be due to the fact that African Americans have higher rates of high blood pressure, diabetes, and obesity. Increased rates of poverty and poor access to health care may also contribute.

Change What You Can

The first step in reducing the risk factors of the person in your care is identifying them. Apply the list of risk factors to this person. If you find that they have risk factors that can't be modified (age, race, gender, heredity), then start modifying all of the risk factors that you can (weight, activity, smoking, blood pressure). Implement a diet, exercise, and weight-loss program that works for them. Make sure to check with your doctor before starting an exercise program because he or she might want to limit what the person in your care can do.

NOTE It is important that the person in your care take as much responsibility as possible for making and maintaining these changes. An individual is more likely to change his lifestyle and stick with them, if he is a partner in the process. Sometimes people become angry and resist changes if they feel they are being forced into them and feel they were not part of the decision.

Medication

The person in your care will be on medications for his heart failure for the rest of his life. Be sure to fill the prescription on time (to avoid running out) and be diligent that the person in your care takes it *exactly* as directed. At first, you will have to make medication management a priority, but after awhile, it will become a habit like brushing your teeth.

NOTE More than half of all prescriptions are taken incorrectly or not at all. No drug can work as expected if it's not taken as directed. Heart failure medication must be taken as prescribed and NOT just when someone has symptoms.

Blood Pressure

You or the care receiver need to monitor his or her blood pressure on a daily basis or take it prior to each dose of medication that could lower his blood pressure. If your care receiver has low blood pressure, this would **not** be uncommon. However, if your care receiver has low blood pressure and is symptomatic (dizzy or lightheaded), contact their doctor immediately to discuss the symptoms. DO NOT stop taking any prescribed medication without the approval of his/her doctor.

Cholesterol and Salt Consumption

Because cholesterol is a major factor in coronary artery disease, it is important to get it checked both in yourself and the person in your care. High numbers may be reduced through appropriate diet, regular exercise, and weight loss. If that doesn't work, check with the doctor about cholesterol-lowering drugs.

The typical American diet is very high in sodium. Even if no salt is added during cooking, most people still consume too much sodium because most processed foods, such as frozen dinners, boxed noodles, and canned soups and vegetables, are high in sodium. When an individual consumes too much sodium, extra fluid builds up in the body, which causes the heart to work harder. So it is very important to look at labels when grocery shopping to avoid foods/products high in sodium. *(See **Chapter 15, Diet Nutrition, and Exercise** for more information on dietary restrictions.)*

> **NOTE** You may hear health care providers talk about low-sodium diet or low-salt diet and wonder if they are the same or whether they are two different diets. There is no difference between the two, doctors and nurses use the terms *sodium* and *salt* to mean the same thing.

Diabetes

People with diabetes are more than twice as likely to develop heart failure as people without diabetes. Make sure that you and the person in your care are tested for diabetes and alter your lifestyle accordingly.

Depression

Roughly four percent of the general population experiences depression. People with heart failure and their caregivers have depression at much higher rates than the general public. Both the caregiver and the person in their care need to be aware of mood changes in themselves and each other. In *Chapter 14, Special Challenges,* we outline why it is so important to make efforts to prevent depression and to treat it if and when it develops. One important reason to treat depression is that it is associated with increased risk of cardiovascular disease. This affects both you and the person in your care. Depression is a real disease, not a character flaw. Depressed people can not just snap their fingers and make depression go away.

If depression is not treated, it gets worse and causes more problems. Relationships can suffer, and it becomes difficult to take care of yourself. People who feel depressed often isolate themselves, which only makes them feel worse. Fortunately, depression responds well to treatment. It can be difficult to talk about depression, either about your own depressed feelings or the feelings of the person in your care. Nonetheless, it is important to have that talk with a health care provider and then discuss a plan. A primary care doctor or cardiologist can offer ideas about treating depression.

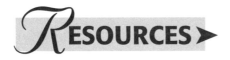

RESOURCES ►

Heart Failure Society of America, Inc.
Box 358
420 Delaware Street, SE
Minneapolis, MN 55455
Phone: (612) 626-3864
www.hfsa.org

American Heart Association
7272 Greenville Avenue
Dallas, TX 75231
Phone: (214) 373-6300 or
1-800-AHA-USA1
www.amhrt.org

National Heart, Lung and Blood Institute
National Institutes of Health
31 Center Drive, Bldg. 31, Room 5A52
Baltimore, MD 20892
Phone: (301) 496-4236
www.nhlbi.nih.gov

American Diabetes Association
1701 North Beauregard Street
Alexandria, VA 22311
http://diabetes.org

Publications

Martensson, J., Dracup, K., Canary, C., & Fridlund, B. (2003). Living with Heart Failure: Depression and Quality of Life in Patients and Spouses. *The Journal of Heart and Lung Transplantation, 22,* (4), 460–467.

Hooley, P. J. (2005). The Relationship of Quality of Life, Depression, and Caregiver Burden in Outpatients with Congestive Heart Failure. *Congestive Heart Failure, 11,* (6), 303–310.

Assessing and Diagnosing Heart Failure

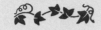

Assessing and Diagnosing Heart Failure

*L*ike many other conditions, heart failure is diagnosed by considering several types of information including: symptoms (shortness of breath, tiredness and fluid buildup), a detailed medical history, physical examination, and other diagnostic testing. This work-up identifies the presence of diseases and conditions that can cause heart failure. It also rules out any other explanation for the patient's symptoms and determines the amount of damage to the pumping ability of the person's heart.

Medical and Family History

The doctor will obtain a personal and family medical history. It helps to know if there are other diseases or conditions that can contribute to heart failure, such as diabetes, coronary heart disease, high blood pressure, a recent viral illness and smoking or alcohol use. The doctor will also perform a complete physical examination to look for signs of heart failure. He might ask about types of symptoms the patient has experienced, when they occurred, how long they have had those symptoms and their severity. This information helps the doctor determine the stage of heart failure (*discussed later in this chapter*) and the limitations the patient might have in performing daily activities.

Physical Examination

As mentioned above, when the person in your care goes for a doctor's appointment, the doctor will perform a complete physical examination to look for signs of heart failure. The doctor will listen to the heart for abnormal sounds, to the lungs, for any build-up of fluid, and look for swelling in the feet, ankles, legs, or abdomen as well as for bulging neck veins. Expect that this will be done at every visit.

Tests

In addition to the physical examination and evaluation of symptoms, the doctor may request additional testing in order to fully diagnose the patient's heart failure. Some of the tests your doctor may request are:

Blood Tests

Blood tests are done to evaluate kidney and thyroid function, as well as cholesterol levels and the presence of anemia. A special test, called B-type Natriuretic Peptide (BNP), can also be done. BNP is a substance that is secreted from the lower chambers of the heart in response to changes in pressure that occur when heart failure develops. The level of BNP in the blood increases as heart failure symptoms worsen.

Another special blood test done to check for inflammation in the heart is a highly sensitive C-reactive protein (hs-CRP) assay, which helps find out if a person has an increased chance of having a sudden heart problem, such as a heart attack. Inflammation can damage the inner lining of the arteries and make having a heart attack more likely.

NOTE A person with stable heart failure has a higher BNP level than a person with normal heart function. In addition, a BNP level helps the doctor determine if admission to a hospital is warranted or if more aggressive treatments are needed.

Chest X-ray

A chest x-ray is a picture of the heart and lungs. It can show the size of the heart and whether or not there is fluid build-up around the lungs.

Electrocardiogram (EKG or ECG)

An EKG or ECG looks at the rate and regularity of heartbeat. It records the electrical activity of the heart and can show if there has been a heart attack or if there is thickening in the walls of the heart's lower chambers (ventricles). During this test, sticky patches called electrodes are placed on the patient's chest, legs and arms and are hooked up to an EKG monitor that records the heart's rhythm.

Echocardiogram (or echo)

An echocardiogram is one of the most useful tests for diagnosing heart failure. During an echo, a gel-like substance is put on the chest, and a wand is used to send an ultrasound wave that provides a picture of the moving heart. This test is done to evaluate the size and shape of the heart, its pumping ability and how the valves are working. It also measures the *ejection fraction,* which tells the doctor how much blood is pumped out of the heart with each beat. A normal ejection fraction is greater than 50 percent, which means that over half of the blood volume is pumped out of the heart with each beat.

Cardiac Catheterization

This test involves inserting a small, flexible tube into an artery in either the groin (leg) or arm to reach the heart. This tube is guided to the heart by use of a special x-ray machine. By injecting contrast dye, this study allows the doctor to see inside the coronary arteries to determine if there are any blockages. This is called a **left-heart catheterization** or **coronary angiography**. A **right-heart catheterization** can also be done at the same time if needed. This looks at the function of the heart, and samples of the heart (a biopsy) can also be taken, if needed.

Depending on the patient's condition, the doctor may order other tests. These may include, but are not limited to:

Stress Test

This diagnostic test looks at how the heart responds to stress. It usually involves walking on a treadmill or riding a stationary bike. For patients who cannot perform these activities, medications may be used to put stress on the heart.

Nuclear Scan (MUGA scan)

This test evaluates the heart's pumping function by using a small amount of radioactive tracer injected into the bloodstream.

Stages/Classifications of Heart Failure

To determine how to treat heart failure patients, physicians often assess heart failure according to the New York Heart Association (NYHA) functional classification system. This system relates symptoms to everyday activities and the patient's quality of life. In addition to this system, the American College of Cardiology (ACC) and the American Heart Association (AHA) have developed the "stages of heart failure." These stages help the person in your care understand that heart failure is a progressive condition and can worsen over time.

Both the stages and the classifications can help you and the person in your care understand why lifestyle changes, such as diet and quitting smoking, are needed or why a new medication has been added or why a treatment plan needs to be altered.

 It is important to know that once a particular "stage" of heart failure has been reached, the patient cannot improve and go back to a previous stage. This is not true for classifications, because patients can move both ways on the NYHA functional classification system.

The following table compares the stages and functional classifications of heart failure.

ACC/AHA Stage		NYHA Functional Class	
Stage	Description	Class	Description
A	Patients at high risk of developing heart failure (pre-heart failure). Could include people with diabetes, hypertension, history of drug or alcohol abuse, etc…, but without structural heart disease or symptoms of heart failure.	No comparable functional class	
B	Patients who have developed structural heart disease but have no symptoms of heart failure.	I (No symptoms)	No limitation of physical activity
C	Patients who have current or prior symptoms of heart failure associated with underlying structural heart disease.	II (Mild)	Slight limitation of physical activity. Comfortable at rest, but ordinary physical activity results in being tired, palpitations or shortness of breath.
		III (Moderate)	Marked limitation of physical activity. Comfortable at rest, but a little activity, such as bathing or dressing, results in being tired, palpitations or shortness of breath.
D	Patients with advanced structural heart disease and marked symptoms of heart failure at rest despite maximal medical therapy. May require specialized therapies like heart transplant or mechanical-assist devices.	IV (Severe)	Unable to carry out any physical activity without discomfort. Symptoms evident at rest. If any physical activity is undertaken, discomfort is increased.

Signs and Symptoms of Heart Failure

Heart failure can cause many symptoms, and some symptoms are more serious than others. It is important that you and the person in your care are able to recognize these symptoms and know when to call your doctor or nurse versus when to call 911 for urgent help. Noticing these early changes and taking the appropriate steps to manage them may help prevent a more urgent problem from developing or even prevent a hospital stay.

NOTE It is important to tell the doctor or nurse about any changes in the patient's condition or symptoms, even if they seem small. Small changes may not seem urgent to you, but they can get worse if ignored.

You should notify your doctor or nurse if the person in your care is experiencing the following symptoms – do not wait for the symptoms to become an urgent problem:

- A weight gain **or** loss of more than 3 pounds in a 1–2 day period, or 4–5 pounds in a 3–5 day period

- Swelling in the legs, feet, hands, or abdomen (Rings, shoes or pants may feel tight with mild swelling.)

- A persistent cough or chest congestion

- A loss of appetite or nausea and vomiting

- Increasing fatigue (feeling tired) or a sudden decrease in her ability to do normal activities.

- A feeling of fullness or bloating in her stomach

- Confusion

- Shortness of breath (that is new, becomes worse or occurs more often, or if it occurs at rest or wakes her from sleep). Observe the number of pillows the person in your care uses to keep from being short of breath during the night. If this increases, report it to the doctor because this might indicate that her heart failure is worsening.

- Dizziness or lightheadedness or a feeling as if she might pass out

- Decreased urination or dark urine

- Chest pain or discomfort during activity that is relieved with rest

- A newly irregular heartbeat or a faster heart rate than normal

- Low blood pressures (especially after taking medications)

- Any other symptom that causes the person in your care stress or concern

These symptoms are early signs that fluid may be building up or that the heart failure of the person in your care is worsening or not responding to treatment. If they have any of these symptoms, it is important to tell the doctor or nurse about them. They may be able to help decrease these symptoms or get rid of them.

 It is also very important to let the doctor or nurse know if the person in your care has new symptoms after a new medication is started. The person in your care may not be able to tolerate the medicine or dose prescribed, so the doctor will need to make changes that allow the person in your care to tolerate the medication better.

If the person in your care is experiencing extreme difficulty, call an ambulance immediately. Some people with heart failure have a sudden change in their symptoms that requires immediate attention, like sudden onset of shortness of breath or a fainting spell. If you feel it is urgent, DO NOT WAIT for the doctor or nurse to get back to you, CALL 911 immediately.

> **NOTE** Fatigue (feeling tired) is a common symptom for patients with heart failure. Surprisingly, the best treatment for fatigue is physical activity. However, remember the person in your care should not do too much at one time. He should schedule things at varying times throughout the day, so he can alternate between rest and activity. See ▭ Chapter 12, *Activities of Daily Living,* for more details.

Signs and Symptoms of Heart Attack and Stroke

In addition to heart failure symptoms, it is important that you and the person in your care are able to recognize the signs and symptoms of heart attack and stroke. The quicker a person having such an event gets to a hospital and receives medical attention, the better her chances of surviving it.

> **NOTE** If you are worried about symptoms the person in your care is experiencing, you should act quickly, be firm and insist that she get help.

Warning Signs of a Heart Attack

Like heart failure symptoms, warning signs of a heart attack can be both sudden and intense or they can start out with mild aches and pains and develop slowly. It is important to be able to recognize these warning signs and report them immediately by calling 911:

- New chest pain or discomfort that lasts longer than 15 minutes and is not relieved by rest or medication

- Discomfort in other areas of the body (jaw, neck, back or arm)

- Breaking out in a cold sweat, nausea/vomiting or light-headedness

- Fainting spell or loss of consciousness

Warning Signs of Stroke

Stroke is a medical emergency, so it is important for you to be able to recognize the warning signs so you can get the person in your care to an emergency room as quickly as possible. Quick treatment is the best way to prevent long-term deficits from a stroke. The quicker you or the person in your care recognizes these symptoms and calls 911, the better chance of avoiding permanent side effects. If the person in your care has *any* of these warning signs, call 911 immediately; do not wait and see if the symptom resolves itself:

- Sudden weakness or numbness of the face, arm, or leg, especially on one side of the body

- Sudden confusion, trouble speaking or understanding speech

- Sudden trouble seeing in one eye or both

- Sudden trouble walking, dizziness, or loss of balance or coordination

- Sudden, severe headache with no reason

An accurate diagnosis is the important first step in learning to live with and manage heart failure. Once diagnosed, then ongoing assessment and treatment can occur. Treatment will change as the disease progresses. How the person in your care feels from day to day will also vary. It is important to keep the doctor updated about symptoms and to respond immediately to any sudden or worrisome changes.

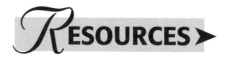 **RESOURCES ➤**

National Heart, Lung and Blood Institute
National Institutes of Health
31 Center Drive, Bldg. 31, Room 5A52
Baltimore, MD 20892
Phone: (301) 496-4236
www.nhlbi.nih.gov

American Heart Association
7272 Greenville Avenue
Dallas, TX 75231
Phone: (214) 373-6300 or
1-800-AHA-USA1
www.amhrt.org

Heart Failure Society of America, Inc.
Box 358
420 Delaware Street, SE
Minneapolis, MN 55455
Phone: (612) 626-3864
www.hfsa.org

American College of Cardiology
www.acc.org/clinical/guidelines/failure

Treatment of Heart Failure

Treatment of Heart Failure

*A*s discussed earlier, heart failure is a serious chronic condition that can change or shorten a person's life. Advances in treatment can help slow, stop or in some cases improve the symptoms of heart failure. However, heart failure is unpredictable and different for each person, so even with the best medical care and treatment, it may continue to get worse over time.

Medical Options

The goals of treating heart failure are the same for all individuals:

- to treat the underlying cause,

- to improve symptoms and quality of life,

- to stop heart failure from getting worse, and

- to prolong life.

In order to do this effectively, a doctor might ask the person in your care to make some lifestyle changes along with prescribed medical treatment.

Lifestyle Changes

Diet

Diet is one lifestyle change that is very important in the treatment plan of heart failure patients. Following a low-salt diet and limiting the amount of fluids are vital in decreasing the symptoms of heart failure. Following this diet may prevent a hospital admission as well. For more detailed information on dietary restriction for the heart failure patient, refer to *Chapter 15-Diet, Nutrition, and Exercise.*

Exercise

Participating in daily activity may be challenging for the heart failure patient. Even if physical activity is limited, moving a little each day is still very important. It is common for a person with a cardiac condition to feel frightened about activity. However, it is still vital for him to participate in some sort of activity, such as bathing and dressing, so he can maintain mobility and independence. Something as simple as brushing his teeth and combing his hair can be beneficial.

 NOTE You can also get a prescription for participating in cardiac rehabilitation programs from your physician. For more detailed information on exercise for the heart failure patient, refer to *Chapter 15-Diet, Nutrition, and Exercise.*

Medications

Like most diseases and conditions, medications will be prescribed by your care receiver's physician to help treat their heart failure. The types and doses of medication will likely be adjusted over time. There are ongoing medical improvements in treating heart failure, so new medications may be added. The doctor will work with your care receiver to try and establish the best medication regimen to help relieve symptoms and improve function.

NOTE Remember, medications are prescribed to help improve heart failure symptoms and to help slow the heart failure process; they will NOT cure heart failure. If the person in your care is feeling better, this does NOT mean they should stop any medications unless previously discussed with her physician.

NOTE As with all medications, it is important to read the inserts provided with each medication for side effects and contraindications. If you observe any of these side effects developing, report them to the physician, PRIOR to stopping the medication.

Types of Medications

There are many types of medications prescribed to treat heart failure. The following list includes both the name of the generic compound and the name under which is marketed in parenthesis.

- *Angiotension Converting Enzyme (ACE) Inhibitors*

  Medication Names: Captopril (Capoten), Lisinopril (Prinivil, Zestril), Fosinopril (Monopril), Enalapril (Vasotec), Quinapril (Accupril), Trandolapril (Mavik), and Ramipril (Altace).

  These medications helps reduce the strain on the heart by lowering blood pressure by dilating (opening) the blood vessels. These drugs can also decrease the risk of heart attack.

- *Angiotensin II Receptor Blockers (ARB)*

  Medication Names: Losartan (Cozaar), Candesartan (Atacand), Telmisartan (Micardis), Valsartan (Diovan) and Irbesartan (Avapro).

  These medications also helps reduce the strain on the heart by lowering blood pressure by dilating (opening) the blood vessels.

- *Beta-Blockers*

  Medication Names: Bisoprolol (Zebeta), Metoprolol (Metoprolol, Toprol-XL), Carvedilol (Coreg).

  These medications helps slow the heart rate and lower blood pressure to decrease the workload on the heart. Over time, beta-blockers may help improve the heart's pumping ability.

- *Hydralazine/Nitrate Combination*

  Medication Names: Isosorbide Dinitrate (Dilatrate-SR, Iso-Bid, Isonate, Isorbid, Isordil, Isotrate, Sorbitrate), Isosorbide Mononitrate (Imdur), Hydralazine (Apresoline), and Hydralazine with Isosorbide Dinitrate (BiDil).

  The combination of Hydralazine (opens arteries) and a nitrate (opens veins) is used for patients who are unable to tolerate taking an ACE inhibitor or an ARB.

- *Digoxin (Digitalis)*

  Medication Names: Digoxin (Lanoxin, Lanoxicaps), Digitoxin (Crystodigin).

  This medication causes the heart to beat more strongly and to pump more blood.

- *Aldosterone Inhibitors*

  Medication Names: Spironolactone (Aldactone) and Eplerenone (Inspra).

  These medications protect the heart by blocking a certain chemical (aldosterone) in the body that causes salt and fluid to buildup. This medicine also helps the heart get stronger.

- *Diuretics (a.k.a water pills)*

  Medication Names: Furosemide (Lasix), Bumetanide (Bumex), Torsemide (Demadex), Metolazone (Zaroxolyn) and Hydrochlorotiazide (Esidrix).

  These medications help decrease the fluid that builds up in the lungs, abdomen, feet or ankles via the kidneys. Getting rid of this fluid makes it easier for the heart to pump and for the patient to breath.

- *Anti-Arrhythmics*

  Medication Names: Flecainide (Tambocor), Amiodarone (Cordarone/Pacerone), Mexilitine (Mexitil), Procainimide (Procanbid/Pronestyl), Propafenone (Rythmol), and Sotalol (Betapace).

  These medications help treat abnormal heart rhythms. They can also help reduce some of the symptoms caused by the abnormal heart rhythms.

- *Anticoagulants*

  Medication Names: Coumadin (Warfarin).

  Some people with heart failure have irregular heartbeats or other problems, putting them at risk of developing blood clots. Anticoagulants (also known as blood thinners) are prescribed to help prevent blood clots.

- *Supplements*

  Potassium or magnesium

  Some diuretics (see above) that help decrease fluid build-up also cause the body to lose potassium and magnesium. These minerals help the heart beat correctly, and sometimes a physician prescribes supplements to make sure there are enough of these minerals in the body.

Tips for Taking Medications

- Take all medications as prescribed.

- In case of emergency, always carry an updated list of medications, their dosage and how often and when they are taken.

- Use a pillbox for medications. Fill the pillbox on a weekly basis so they will always be ready.

- Be sure to get refills on medications **before** they run out.

- Give medications at the same time each day. Remember to give diuretics in the morning to avoid frequent urination throughout the night. If a diuretic is prescribed twice daily, give the evening dose before 5 P.M.

- Do not skip doses, but if a dose is missed, do not double up on it the next time it is due.

- Check with the physician **before** adding any over-the-counter medications. They may interact with some of the heart failure medications.

- If a medication needs to be taken several times throughout the day, ask the doctor if there is a similar medication that can be taken only once or twice daily.

- If the person in your care experiences dizziness or other side effects after taking a prescribed medication, do not stop giving that medication without talking to the doctor.

Compliance

Changing habits is not easy, but it is very important to follow through with the recommendations and treatment plan made by the health care team. These lifestyle changes and medications can decrease symptoms of the person in your care and the frequency of hospital stays. Complying with the doctors' recommendation and treatment plan can improve the quality of life for the person in your care. If you or the person in your care has concerns about the treatment plan, talk to the doctor, nurse or social worker. They may be able to help by—

- suggesting classes to learn about dietary restrictions,

- prescribing less expensive or less cumbersome medications or

- connecting you or the person in your care with other heart failure patients who can demonstrate other ways to follow through with the treatment plan. (See *Resources section at end of chapter*.)

Surgical Options

As heart failure progresses, medical therapy alone may not be enough to control worsening symptoms. As heart failure becomes more severe, the person in your care may be hospitalized from time to time, or they may need to see another type of specialist, such as a cardiologist with specialized training in the diagnosis and treatment of heart rhythm problems (an electrophysiologist), a surgeon, or a transplant cardiologist or surgeon (a doctor who implants ventricular assist devices [VAD] and does heart transplants). These specialists may suggest additional treatments or therapy beyond medical treatment. This therapy might include the following procedures.

Percutaneous Coronary Intervention (PCI)/Stenting

This procedure is used for coronary artery disease patients who may have persistent angina despite medical therapy or who can't undergo surgery. In this procedure, a physician uses a flexible plastic catheter with a balloon at the end to open narrowed arteries in the heart (also called *angioplasty*). The procedure usually involves placing a metal stent to hold the artery open, which restores blood flow to the heart muscle.

Surgery (Coronary Artery Bypass Graft [CABG]), Valve Surgery or Left Ventricular Reconstruction (Dor procedure)

Heart failure may be caused by blocked coronary arteries, stretched-out or blocked valves or a scarred area in the left ventricle of the heart, as discussed in Chapter 1. If a person's heart failure is caused by one of these medical conditions, the physician may suggest surgery to "fix" these conditions. Though undergoing surgery has increased risks for the heart failure patient, new procedures and medications are available to decrease these risks, and the ultimate goal of surgery is to decrease a heart failure patient's symptoms.

Implantable Cardioverter Defibrillator (ICD)/Biventricular pacemaker (BIV/PPM or CRT)

A person with heart failure may develop arrhythmias or dysrhythmias, which are abnormal heart beats that cause the heart to pump inefficiently. If this is a concern for the person in your care, his physician may refer him to a cardiologist with specialized training in treating heart rhythm problems (called an *electrophysiologist* or EP doctor). This specialist may recommend implanting an ICD (implantable cardioverter defibrillator), which is an electronic device that monitors a person's heart rhythm. If the ICD detects an abnormal rhythm, it delivers a small shock to the heart to return it to a normal rhythm. The EP doctor may suggest another therapy, called a BiVentricular pacemaker or CRT (cardiac resynchronization therapy). This device is designed to help the right and left ventricles pump together. CRT is known to improve symptoms associated with heart failure, but not all heart failure patients qualify for this therapy.

Mechanical Heart Pump

A person with severe heart failure, or someone who's medical regimen is failing to control his heart failure symptoms, may be considered for a mechanical heart pump. This special device is placed inside the body to help pump blood. There are several types of mechanical heart pumps. Some people who undergo insertion of a mechanical heart pump may also be considered for a heart transplant.

Heart Transplant

This is a surgery that replaces a failing heart with a healthy heart from someone who has recently died. Transplantation is usually the last resort for persons who continue to worsen when all other treatments have failed.

There are a number of things that the care receiver can do to help manage heart failure; diet, exercise, compliance with medications and doctor's recommendations. In addition to adherence to these recommendations a number of medical treatment options are available. The treatment options for heart failure continue to change and it is important to talk with the physician about new and possibly helpful treatment options for your loved one.

Cardiac Health Improvement and Rehabilitation Program (CHIRP)

Your doctor may encourage the person in your care to participate in a hospital's cardiac rehabilitation program. A cardiac rehabilitation program is designed to help the patient exercise safely and maintain a heart-healthy lifestyle. Most programs generally include:

• Exercise training that helps the person in your care learn how to exercise safely, strengthen their muscles and increase stamina. All exercise programs are tailored to each person's individual ability and needs.

• Education

• Changing risk factors (such as diet)

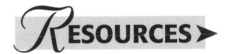 **ESOURCES ➤**

American Heart Association
7272 Greenville Avenue
Dallas, TX 75231
Phone: (214) 373-6300 or
1-800-AHA-USA1
www.amhrt.org

The American Association of Cardiovascular and Pulmonary Rehabilitation (AACVPR)
http://www.aacvpr.org/certification/program_cert_search.cfm
Offers a list of available cardiac rehabilitation programs in all states

Heart Failure Society of America, Inc.
Box 358
420 Delaware Street, SE
Minneapolis, MN 55455
Phone: (612) 626-3864
www.hfsa.org

American Dietetic Association
www.eatright.org
(800) 366-1655
Call weekdays 10:00 a.m. to 5:00 p.m. EST to locate a registered dietitian in your area.

Area Agency on Aging or the Cooperative Extension Service
Your local office offers free counseling by a registered dietitian.

Meals-on-Wheels
www.mealcall.org/ or www.mowaa.org/
Check with your local Department of Aging or a county Department of Human Services
This organization provides nutritious meals delivered to the home.

MyPyramid
www.mypyramid.gov
This replaces the old Food Guide Pyramid. This is a very interactive site designed to help patients and caregivers make healthy choices consistent with the latest dietary guidelines.

Mended Hearts
1-800-AHA-USA1 or 1-800-242-8721
www.mendedhearts.org
This is a nationwide patient support organization for people with heart disease, their families, medical professionals and other interested people.

Web site:
http://www.methodistmd.org/pdf/living_well_with_heart_failure.pdf
Download an excellent twenty-eight page brochure explaining heart failure in simple terms.

Is Home Care for You?

Is Home Care for You?

The need to provide care for another person arises for many reasons. Often, the person who needs care does not realize it, and family members must step in to help make decisions. One of those decisions involves who the caregiver will be and where care will be provided. The choices can be difficult unless you know what to consider.

When one member of the family becomes disabled, roles within the family often change. A person who took care of the family in the past or was the income provider may become dependent, while another person in the family takes on added, often unfamiliar responsibilities. For a single person, the changes may involve a new dependence on non-family members. Just the word "dependence" can cause unpleasant feelings. Being able to talk openly about fears, anxiety, frustration, and doubts can be very helpful in dealing well with these new facts of life.

Discuss chronic care needs with the person's medical team to learn what treatments, adjustments and other changes may be necessary. For some people, training to provide medical treatments, advice on coping with the challenges of chronic illness, and some long-range financial planning will be enough. For others, in-home personal assistance is the best option. Sometimes a nursing home or assisted living center is the better choice for everyone involved.

In making the decision for home care, it is important to be realistic about what the person in your care needs, and what you, the caregiver, can provide in terms of time, kinds of care, and financial responsibility. For example, deciding to hire an in-home attendant may be necessary if the primary caregiver works full time. Before this happens, it's important to look at the financial and emotional issues that go along with this decision.

Caregivers need to think about important issues such as independence, privacy, and the financial effect of hiring in-home help. Then the caregiver needs to talk to the person with the illness and others living in the home about these issues. How will the family pay for in-home help and how will it find the right person(s) or agency?

*Before a person can be hired, the family needs to look at what kind of care is needed: **medical** (symptom management, occupational or physical therapies, etc.), **personal care** (bathing, dressing, using the bathroom, etc.), **homemaking** (shopping, errands, laundry, housecleaning), or **companionship** (social outlets, safety issues, etc.).*

Your Support System

Sometimes children take on major household and personal care duties when a parent has disability. While it is positive for children to take on household jobs and tasks, their needs must be carefully balanced with the amount and level of caregiving they are expected to provide. Children, younger than 18, are not equipped to handle the stress of being the main or primary caregiver. They should never be in charge of a parent's medical treatments or daily functions such as helping with the bathroom.

Family and friends can help. The first step is to let friends and family know that their help is needed and welcomed. Friends often worry that offering help might seem like meddling, especially when things seem to be going well.

Knowing What Level of Care Is Needed

Before you take on the demanding job of home care, decide what level of care you must provide. Do you need to give:

- minimum assistance?

- moderate assistance?

- maximum assistance?

In order to decide what level of care is needed, you must understand the person's condition and needs in the areas of daily care and health. Generally, these needs fall into two broad groups:

Activities of Daily Living (ADLs) are activities such as eating, bathing, dressing, taking medicine, and going to the toilet.

Instrumental Activities of Daily Living (IADLs) are activities that are important to independence, such as cooking, shopping, housekeeping, getting to the doctor, paying bills, and managing money.

Things to look for in deciding the overall level of care needed are the person's—

- ability to get from bed to wheelchair without help
- ability to move without help in wheelchair or walker
- ability to manage bladder and bowel
- ability to carry out the basic activities of daily living
- ability to call for help
- degree of sight and hearing impairment
- degree of confusion

Also, consider emotional conditions that might require advanced or special levels of care:

- depression
- a need to be with other people or to have privacy
- homesickness

After giving some thought to the level of care that might be needed and the person's condition, abilities, and emotional state, try to place the person you might care for in one of these categories:

Minimum Assistance—This person is basically independent, can handle most household chores and personal care, and needs help with only one or two activities of daily living.

Moderate Assistance—This person needs help with three or more activities of daily living, such as bathing, cooking, or shopping.

Maximum Assistance—This person is unable to care for himself or herself, requires total assistance, and must be placed in a nursing home if no skilled caregiver is available in the home. Care is often provided by professionals, either in the home through home service agencies or in foster care homes, assisted living facilities, or nursing homes. At this level, serious problems are a real possibility.

Deciding Whether Home Care Is Possible

When a person has a chronic condition or a terminal illness, daily long-term skilled help with health and personal needs may be in order. Whatever level of care is needed, it can take place in three settings:

- the person's own home

- your home

- residential care facilities, such as a foster care home, assisted living, or a skilled nursing facility

Home Care Considerations

Whether care will take place in your home or in the home of the person who needs care, the following factors must be considered:

- Is there enough room for both the person and items such as a wheelchair, walker, bedside toilet, and lift?

- How accessible is the home if walkers or wheelchairs are used?

- Is a doctor, nurse, or specialist available to supervise care when needed?

- Is there a hospital emergency unit close by?

- Is the home environment safe and supportive and does it allow for some independence?

- Is money available to hire additional help?

- Is the person in question willing to have a caregiver in the home?

- Can the caregiver manage this role along with other family and personal responsibilities?

Things That Must Be Provided

- medication

- meals

- personal care

- housecleaning

- shopping

- transportation

- companionship

- accessibility (wheelchair ramps, support railings, and changes to the bath and shower stall)

Benefits of Home Care

An already positive and supportive relationship may be strengthened by the experience.

- The relationship between the caregiver and the person in care can grow stronger.

- A great deal of money can be saved on health care costs.

Why Home Care May Not Be Possible

- financial reasons (inadequate health insurance to cover the cost of home nursing)

- family limits (lack of time or money)

- too many physical and emotional demands on the caregiver

- the person's complex medical condition

- the home's physical layout

- the person's desire to live independently of family

Possible Hazards of Home Care

- Possible lack of freedom for the caregiver.

- Caregiver duties may affect the caregiver's job, career, hobbies, and personal life.

- There may be less time for family members, and the caregiver's family relationships may suffer.

- Children in the home may need to be quieter.

- There may be less time for religious activities and volunteer work.

- Friends and family may criticize the caregiver's efforts and offer unwelcome advice.

- The caregiver may often be awakened during the night.

- The caregiver may feel unable to control life's events and may suffer from depression, worry, anger, regrets, guilt, and stress.

- Instead of being grateful, the person receiving care may display unpleasant changes in attitude.

- He may react to constant daily irritations by lashing out at the caregiver.

- The caregiver may begin to fear the time when he may be dependent on someone for care.

- The caregiver may feel obliged to spend personal funds on caregiving.

- The caregiver may become physically ill and emotionally drained.

Outside Help

One of the biggest pitfalls in caregiving is trying to do it all yourself. But other help is available and should be called on whenever possible. That help includes:

- support groups

- day care and respite care, which provide relief for the caregiver

- organizations providing respite care

- pastoral counseling services

- parish nurses

- medical services provided by professionals, such as nurses and therapists

- personal services for the person in your care, such as grooming or dressing, provided by home health aides

Checklist **The Ideal Caregiver**

The ideal caregiver is—

✓ emotionally and physically capable of handling the work

✓ able to share duties and responsibilities with other willing family members

✓ able to plan solutions and solve problems instead of withdrawing under stress

✓ able to speak in a simple and clear way

✓ comfortable giving and receiving help

✓ trained for the level of care required

✓ able to handle unpleasant tasks such as changing diapers, bathing, or cleaning bed sores

✓ in good health and has energy, skill, and the ability to adapt

✓ able to cope with anger and frustration

✓ able to afford respite (back-up) care when necessary

✓ able to speak to and understand the care receiver

✓ able to make this person feel useful and needed

✓ valued by other family members

✓ able to adjust to the future needs and wishes of the person in care

✓ aware of other care options and willing to explore them

If you have most of these traits, you may be a good candidate to provide home care. However, consider the list called "Possible Hazards of Home Care" (earlier in this chapter) and be honest with yourself about your ability to cope.

- community home health services on a fee basis, such as Visiting Nurse Associations (📖 See ***Getting In-Home Help,*** Chapter 7)

- social worker's provided through the Visiting Nurse Associations or a home health care agency

Supportive Housing and Care Options

If you believe that home care is not practical for you, many other options exist. Good programs foster independence, dignity, privacy, a very high level of functioning, and connections with the community. However, people who have lived independently all their lives may not be suited to live in groups, and those who are mentally alert or are younger may be very unhappy living with people who suffer from dementia.

Keep the above factors in mind when you check out the following:

- **Independent Living Options**—apartment buildings, condos, retirement communities, and single-family homes

- **Semi-independent Living Options**—places that offer the same benefits as independent living but also include meal service and housekeeping as part of the monthly fee, provide help with personal care, keep track of health and medications, and provide special diets. These options are frequently offered in assisted living facilities and group homes.

- **Skilled Care Facilities**—nursing homes

States use different names for care facilities. The services can also vary, so it is important to check with the facility and each state's licensing agency to confirm exactly which services are offered. For example, in Wyoming, assisted living allows people who are unrelated to share a room. In some other places, living spaces are not shared, except by personal choice.

A Closer Look at the Options

House Sharing—for people who are fully independent

- Two or more unrelated people live together, each with a private bedroom.

- All living areas are shared.

- Chores and expenses are shared.

- Personal-assistant services may be shared.

Group Homes or Adult Foster Care Homes—homes in residential neighborhoods for people whose needs vary, from assistance with individual services to dependent residents with increased nursing services

- Care is given to small groups of people in the primary caregiver's home or with a live-in resident manager/caregiver.

- The home is privately run and provides private or shared rooms with meals, housekeeping, personal care (such as bathing and dressing), keeping track of medication, safety supervision, and some transportation.

- Rates vary according to individual care needs, and Medicaid funding is often available for repayment to those who qualify.

- Staff are qualified and facilities are licensed according to the level of services offered, which can include housekeeping, laundry, personal care assistance, bathing, dressing, grooming, and management of medication and other medical needs, such as injections or inability to control bladder and bowel.

 Some states do not license, inspect, or keep watch over adult foster care homes. Before selecting one, call your local Area Agency on Aging or the state or county Department of Health to see if any complaints have been filed against the home you are considering.

Assisted Living Facilities—for moderate assistance to those who are frail and usually require assistance with activities of daily living

- Each person lives in his or her own apartment.

- An emergency staff is available 24 hours a day.

- Monthly charges are based on the level of service needed.

- Activities such as games, hobbies, crafts, and music are offered.

- Meals, housekeeping, medication management, and nursing assessment are provided.

- Transportation and access to medical services can be arranged.

 There is no national control over these facilities but there is state licensing and regulation. For information on a specific facility, call the ombudsman in your state or the state agency that licenses the facility. (An ombudsman is someone who looks into complaints made by individuals.)

Continuing Care Retirement Communities—for people who want a range of services from independent living to nursing home care

- These facilities provide a lifetime contract for care.

- They provide or offer meals and can handle special diets.

- They offer housekeeping, scheduled transportation, emergency help, personal care, and activities for fun and learning.

- Many retirement communities require entrance fees that can vary quite a bit.

- They also have monthly fees ranging from several hundred to several thousand dollars.

- Some provide home health care and nursing home care without extra fees.

- Some charge extra for nursing unit residents.

Nursing Homes—for people who require continuous and ongoing nursing assistance or monitoring

Nursing homes typically offer three levels of care:

- **Custodial**—minimal nursing, but help with hygiene, meals, dressing, etc.

- **Intermediate**—help for those who cannot live alone but do not need 24-hour skilled nursing care

- **Skilled Nursing**—intensive 24-hour skilled nursing care

Hospice care is available in all settings as a covered benefit under Medicare. It is also covered for those who receive Medicaid in states that offer hospice coverage under their Medicaid program.

Financing Options

The choice of the right housing option may depend on financing available:

- **Personal Resources** are the most common way to pay.

- **Private Insurance** is helpful, but some policies limit the length and type of benefits and have waiting periods or other limits.

- **Medicare** is for those 65 and older or for people who have been declared disabled by the Social Security Administration. Medicare partially pays for up to 100 days in a skilled nursing care facility after a qualifying related hospitalization of more than three days in a row (not including the day the person leaves the hospital). The financing of hospice care is a separate benefit under Medicare.

- **Medicaid** partially pays for services, including assisted living services in some states, to those who are aged, blind, or have disabilities and have limited financial resources. It is also a major payer for nursing home care.

- **Medigap** policies cover gaps in coverage and may be in place to pay Medicare coinsurance. (See **Paying for Care,** Chapter 8)

Points to Review Before Signing a Contract or Lease

Although it is hard to know what problems may arise in a care setting, it is extremely important to take the following steps before signing any legal papers:

- Find out who owns the facility and review the owner's financial status.

- Ask for a copy of the contract and review it with an attorney or financial advisor.

Checklist **Review Before Deciding on a Facility**

✓ Is a trial period allowed to be sure a person is happy with the facility?

✓ Will the facility refund deposits or entrance fees if the resident dies, chooses to leave, or is asked to leave?

✓ Can a resident choose his or her own apartment? Can personal furniture be used?

✓ Are there younger residents at the facility?

✓ If the person must be away for a short time (even for a hospital stay), will the same apartment be available when he or she returns? Is there a reduced rate during long absences?

✓ If the person marries, can the couple live in the same apartment?

✓ Can the staff handle special diets? Are meal menus posted?

✓ Is transportation provided?

✓ How many people are on staff and how much training have they had?

✓ How often and for what reasons can staff enter the apartment?

✓ Can the resident see his or her own doctor? Who gives out the medications?

✓ Is physical therapy available within the facility?

✓ Is the facility licensed to deal with a resident whose health gets worse or must the person leave if, for example, he or she can no longer walk or begins arguing or fighting with others?

✓ How are decisions made when a person must be moved to another part of the facility?

✓ Is there a 30-day-notice provision for ending the agreement?

✓ Does the facility take Medicare?

✓ Will the facility let a resident "spend down" his or her assets and go on Medicaid?

- Do not rely on spoken promises. Make sure the contract is geared to the resident's needs.

- Read the state inspection report on the facility.

- Read all the rules and policies of the facility that are not in the contract.

- Ask to see the facility's license.

Things You Should Know About Facilities

Residents' Rights

General Rights—Residents maintain all their rights guaranteed under the U.S. Constitution, including the right to vote. In addition, they can receive visitors, voice their concerns, form resident councils, and enjoy informed consent, privacy, and freedom of choice.

Privacy—In some cases, a resident may have a roommate. However, residents' rooms are considered private, and staff must knock before entering. Also, residents can have private visits with spouses.

Restraints—Only the resident's doctor may order a restraint as part of a care plan and must state the specific restraint's use and period of use. (Use of restraints is strongly discouraged, although not prohibited.)

Lifestyle Choices—Residents do not have as many choices as they would have at home regarding meal times, menu choices, and times for sleep. However, most facilities try to satisfy residents' needs as much as possible.

Ability to Effect Change—Issues can be brought up to the resident council or the long-term-care ombudsman.

Freedom to Leave—A person chooses to enter a facility and has the right to leave at any time regardless of safety concerns or what the family thinks.

NOTE The following describes general guidelines regarding a resident's rights. To obtain specific rules for a particular state, contact the state agency responsible for licensing the facility.

The Resident's Rights When Leaving a Facility

Depending on the admission agreement, a resident must be given written notice 30 days before being moved. If there is a medical emergency, no written notice is required. Generally, a resident may be moved from a facility for the following reasons:

- The person wants to be moved.

- The person must be moved for his or her own good.

- The person must be moved for the good of other residents.

- The facility is not being paid. (However, someone who runs out of money cannot be moved if Medicaid will pay.)

- The person came into the facility for special care and that care is completed.

- The facility is being closed.

If the person does not want to leave the facility, IMMEDIATELY contact the state agency responsible for licensing the facility and/or Medicaid certification.

If you have questions, call the following:

- the Center for Medicare-Medicaid Services

- the local Senior and Disabled Services Division of the Department of Health and Human Resources

- the long-term-care ombudsman

- the Federal Health Care Financing Administration
- the local Area Agency on Aging

What Family Members and Friends Should Do

- Visit whenever possible.
- Send cards or letters between visits.
- Bring small gifts and approved treats.
- If allowed, walk around with the person when visiting to provide exercise.
- Listen to the resident's complaints.
- Build a good relationship with the staff.
- Plan off-site outings if appropriate.

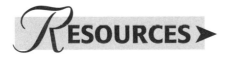

RESOURCES ➤

AARP
601 E Street, NW
Washington, DC 20049
(800) 424-3410
www.aarp.org
Web site provides information on housing and other senior issues.

National Council on Independent Living
1916 Wilson Boulevard, Suite 209
Arlington, VA 22201
(703) 525-3406 (voice)
(703) 525-4153 (tty)
ncil@ncil.org

www.ncil.org
Refers callers to local independent-living centers. Offers publications and advice related to disability issues. Advocates for policy changes.

Assisted Living Facilities and Nursing Homes

American Association of Homes and Services for the Aging
2519 Connecticut Avenue, NW
Washington, DC 20008
(202) 783-2255
(800) 508-9442
www.aahsa.org
Provides information on not-for-profit nursing homes, senior housing facilities, assisted living, and community services. Call for free consumer information brochure.

American Health Care Association/National Center for Assisted Living
1201 L Street, NW
Washington, DC 20005
(202) 842-4444
www.ahca.org
Provides consumer information on services, financing, public policy, nursing facilities, assisted living, and subacute care. Represents more than 10,000 providers of assisted living, nursing care, and subacute care.

Assisted Living Federation of America
11200 Waples Mill Road, Suite 150
Fairfax, VA 22030
(703) 691-8100
www.alfa.org
Offers referrals to local facilities listed by state. Provides free 15-page consumer guide to assisted living.

The Center for Medicare and Medicaid Services has detailed information about the past performance of every Medicare- and Medicaid-certified nursing home in the country. For more information, go to www.medicare.gov, click on Search Tools at the top of the page, and then click on Compare Nursing Homes in Your Area. For a list of **Medicare-certified nursing homes,** call the local office or department on aging.

Respite Services

ARCH National Respite Locator Service
800 Eastowne Drive, Suite 105
Chapel Hill, NC 27514-2204
(919) 490-5577
www.respitelocator.org
Provides caregivers with contact information on respite services in their area.

Eldercare Locator
National Association of Area Agencies on Aging
1730 Rhode Island Avenue, NW, Suite 1200
Washington, DC 20036
(800) 677-1116
www.eldercare.gov
www.aoa.dhhs.gov
Supplies information about many eldercare issues, including respite care. Provides referrals to local respite programs and local Area Agency on Aging.

If you don't have access to the Internet, ask your local library to help you locate a Web site.

For a list of **Medicare Certified Nursing Homes,** call the local Office on Aging.

Using the Health Care Team Effectively

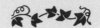

Using the Health Care Team Effectively

*W*hen you care for someone in the home, you must also manage that person's health care. This means choosing a good medical team, keeping costs down, arranging for medical appointments, and getting the best, least expensive medicines. It also means knowing what the insurance rules are and, most important, being an advocate (a supporter) for the person in your care. Include care receiver in decision making as much as possible.

Doctors and nurses can focus on physical diagnosis and may pay less attention to the emotional aspects of care. They may not consider the spiritual aspects of healing. Although you should consult with professionals about the levels of therapy and support needed for the person in your care, you do not have to accept what they suggest or order. Keep asking questions until you completely understand the diagnosis (what is wrong), treatment, and prognosis (likely outcome).

Who Makes Up Your Heart Failure Team?

Heart failure can be challenging to manage, but symptoms can often be controlled if the cardiac patient pays attention to care recommendations. These might include taking medications as prescribed, following a low-salt/sodium diet, and maintaining medical appointments. The person in your care needs to report changes in his condition to the treatment team so that adjustments in care can be made. With advances in heart failure management, patients can now survive many years after they have been diagnosed with this condition. It is important that both you and the person in your care develop a good working relationship with the treatment team. The members of this team will be part of the life of the person in your care for an extended time. Each of the team members has a different job, and it is important that you and the person in your care trust the team. This can take some time to develop. You and the person in your care may feel more comfortable with some of these care providers than others, but for successful management of heart failure, you and the person in your care will need the ongoing care of ALL of the treatment team.

Members of the Heart Failure Team

Several specialists are involved in the care of a heart failure patient. Of course, the first step is to see your **Primary Care Physician.** This doctor can advise on the next step in treatment. This could include additional testing or involve seeing a specialist to manage the patient's heart failure. Some of these specialized physicians may include:

- **Cardiologist**—specializes in the diagnosis, treatment, and prevention of diseases of the heart and blood vessels.

- **Heart Failure Specialist**—a cardiologist who focuses on the diagnosis and treatment of heart failure. This emerging specialty is growing steadily to meet the needs of an aging population in which heart failure is more common.

- **Registered Nurse**—works in collaboration with physician in the treatment and prevention of diseases.

- **Nurse Practitioner**—works in the treatment and prevention of diseases with the collaboration of a physician.

- **Heart Failure Disease Management Clinic**—an out-patient clinic that focuses on the management of heart failure conditions and symptoms. This is a multi-team member clinic consisting of a registered nurse, nurse practitioner, and physician specializing in heart failure.

- **Electrophysiologist (EP) or Heart Rhythm Specialist**—a cardiologist with specialized training in the diagnosis and treatment of heart rhythm problems.

- **Dietitian**—a registered dietitian can provide in-depth, personalized nutrition education and help a patient begin a personal action plan. (See *Chapter 15, Diet, Nutrition, and Exercise*)

- **Physical Therapist**—a health care professional who teaches exercises and physical activities that help condition muscles and restore strength and movement safely, while increasing stamina.

- **Occupational Therapist**—a health care professional who specializes in helping people reach their maximum level of function and independence in all aspects of daily life.

- **Surgeon and/or Transplant Surgeon**—a specialist who does operations on the heart, including implanting ventricular assist devices (VAD) and heart transplantation. (See *Chapter 4, Treatment of Heart Failure, for more detailed information on ventricular assist devices.*)

NOTE A specialist will typically send back full reports to the primary care physician who knows the entire medical history and is a key partner in the long-term management of the heart conditions of the person in your care. Typically, caregivers continue to work with the primary care doctor of the person in their care to manage all aspects of health care.

Choosing a Doctor

Call your local medical or dental society for the names of doctors who specialize in the field in which you seek care. Think about using doctors who are allied with medical schools. They tend to have the most up-to-date information, especially about complicated illnesses.

- Always make sure the doctor is board certified in his or her specialty.

- If the person in your care is enrolled in an HMO, ask if the doctor is planning to change HMOs anytime soon.

- You can contact more than one doctor (for a second opinion). If you are enrolled in Medicare Supplementary Medical Insurance (Part B), Medicare will pay for a second opinion in the same way it pays for other services. After Part B of the deductible has been met, Medicare pays 80 percent of the Medicare-approved amount for a second opinion and will provide the same coverage for a third opinion.

Nurse Practitioners

Seek out a medical practice that incorporates the services of a nurse practitioner or physician assistant. These mid-level practitioners provide health screening, perform physical examinations, order laboratory tests, and prescribe specific medications authorized by the physician. Nurse practitioners also educate patients about staying healthy. Often they are the best-equipped health professionals to educate patients and caregivers about the common problems of chronic illness. Mid-level health care providers usually spend more time with patients and caregivers than the supervising medical specialists in a busy practice.

How to Share in Medical Decisions

In the end, medical decision-making is in the hands of the person receiving care, the doctor, and the caregiver. Learn to take an active role and become an advocate for yourself and for the person in your care. It has been said that a patient is the senior partner in the patient–doctor relationship.

Long-Range Considerations

- Find out how the person in your care feels about treatments that prolong life. Respect these views.

- Help the person receiving care to set up an advance directive and power of attorney for health care. (📖 See **Planning for End-of-Life Care,** Chapter 9)

- Share decisions with the doctor and the care receiver and take responsibility for the treatment and its outcomes.

The Doctor–Patient–Caregiver Relationship

- Be aware that doctors must see more patients per day than they once did.

- Be aware that some doctors may have financial reasons for doing too much or too little for those in their care. Specialists are often the only ones with the training needed to treat a serious or chronic condition, so the doctor may refer the care receiver to a specialist.

- If the relationship with the doctor becomes unfriendly, consider finding a new doctor.

- Respect the doctor's time (you may need to have more than one visit to cover all issues).

- If Medicare is the payer, ask if the doctor accepts Medicare assignment. If not, the difference may have to be paid out of pocket.

Preparing for a Visit to the Doctor

- Be prepared to briefly explain the care receiver's and the family's medical history.

- Take a list of questions in order of importance.

- Prepare a list of any symptoms the person you care for is experiencing.

- Be prepared to ask for written information on the medical situation so you can better understand what the doctor is saying, or bring a small tape recorder.

- You can call the hospital's library or health resource center for help in looking up any questions the doctor does not answer.

 Be sure shots for tetanus, flu, and pneumonia are up-to-date. For those on Medicare, flu and pneumonia shots are covered.

At the Doctor's Office

- Tell the doctor what you hope and expect from the visit and any recommended treatment.

- If the doctor tells you to do something you know you can't do, such as give medication in the middle of the night, ask if there is another treatment and explain why.

- Insist on talking about the level of care that you believe is appropriate and that agrees with the care receiver's wishes.

- Ask about other options for tests, medications, and surgery.

- Ask why tests or treatments are needed and what the risks are.

- Consider all options, including the pros and cons of "watchful waiting."

- Trust your common sense and if you have doubts, get a second opinion.

Checklist Changes to Report to the Doctor

Contact the doctor right away if the following changes occur. Fever may be caused by an infection and should always be reported:

Ability to Move

✓ *falls, even if there is no pain*

✓ *leg pain when walking*

✓ *painful or limited movement (color of skin over painful areas should be reported)*

✓ *inability to move*

Diet

✓ *extreme thirst*

✓ *lack of thirst*

✓ *weight loss or weight gain of 3-5 pounds in a 1-2 day period for no reason*

✓ *loss of appetite*

✓ *pain before or after eating*

✓ *difficulty chewing or swallowing*

✓ *pain in the gums or teeth*

✓ *frequent gum infections*

Behavior

✓ *unusual tiredness or sleepiness*

✓ *unusual actions (arguing, fighting, anger, or withdrawal)*

✓ *seeing or hearing things that aren't there (hallucinations)*

✓ *anxiety*

✓ *increased confusion*

✓ *depression*

✓ *inappropriate or unusual emotions*

Bowel/Bladder

✓ *bowel movements of an odd color, texture, or amount*

✓ *feeling faint during bowel movements*

✓ *vaginal discharge (report color, odor, amount)*

✓ *draining sores or pain in the penis area*

✓ *pain when going to the bathroom (unusual color, amount, or odor)*

✓ *having a decrease in amount or frequency of urination*

✓ *frequent bladder infections*

✓ *blood in the urine*

✓ *pain in the kidney area*

Skin

✓ changes in the color of lips, nails, fingers, and toes

✓ odd skin (color, temperature, texture, bruises)

✓ unusual appearance of surgery incisions

✓ sudden skin rashes (bumps, itching)

✓ pressure sores (bedsores)

Bones, Muscles, and Joints

✓ swelling in the arms and legs or around the eyes

✓ twitching or movement that cannot be controlled

✓ tingling or numbness in hands, feet, and other parts of the body

✓ warm, tender joints

✓ redness in the joints

✓ unusual position of arms, legs, fingers, or toes

Chest

✓ chest pain

✓ rapid pulse

✓ problems with breasts (report lumps, discharge, soreness, or draining)

✓ painful breathing (wheezing, shortness of breath)

✓ unusual cough

✓ unusual saliva or mucus (report color and consistency)

Abdomen

✓ stomach pain or bloating

✓ nausea or vomiting

Head

✓ dizziness (if this occurs, check blood pressure and report any significant changes)

✓ headaches

✓ ear pain, discharge, or change in hearing

✓ eye pain, discharge, redness, blurry vision, or being bothered by light

✓ mouth sores

✓ nose pain (bleeding, bad odor to mucus)

KEEP ASKING QUESTIONS UNTIL YOU ARE SATISFIED. *Doctors and other health care professionals have medical know-how, but only you can explain symptoms. Report exactly, in as few words as possible, any unusual symptoms, changes in condition, and complaints the person has.*

If the Person in Your Care Is Near Death

- Doctors may have limited training in talking about death and the dying process with their patients. Be prepared to begin the conversation yourself.

- If the person in your care wants to die at home, say this clearly to the doctor.

- Be sure that any directives for health care for the person are available and prominently displayed.

Questions to Ask Before Agreeing to Tests, Medications, and Surgery

Before you begin discussing medical treatment with the doctor, explain that the person in your care does not want any unnecessary tests or treatments. Then ask these questions:

- Why is this test needed?

- How long will it take? How soon will the results be in?

 If your doctor recommends a procedure and the HMO refuses to cover it, see Appealing an HMO Decision in Chapter 8, **Paying for Care**.

Questions to Ask the Doctor About Medications

Medications can be costly, confusing to use, and have unwanted side effects. Be sure to ask questions when medicines are prescribed and prescriptions are filled.

- Give the doctor a list of all medications and dosages that the person in your care is now taking, including eye drops, vitamins, and herbal remedies.

- Tell the doctor of any other treatments being used. Sometimes using two or more treatments may be fatal or may keep the new treatment from working.

- Tell the doctor of any allergies or if there are certain foods the person cannot eat (food allergies).

- Understand why each medication is needed and how much it will help the person's condition.

- Ask if pain can be relieved almost completely, and then ask for the medicine that works best.

- Ask how long it takes for the drug to work.

- Find out its side effects.

- Ask if the drug could react with other drugs and what you should do if there are side effects.

- Find out if a change in diet, exercise, reducing stress, or other things can be done.

- If more than one medicine is needed, ask the doctor if they can be taken at the same times each day. If a drug must be taken at a difficult time (for instance, in the middle of the night), ask about another choice.

- Try to find the lowest cost drug. Ask if a generic (nonbrand name) drug or another brand in the same drug class is available at a lower cost.

- Be sure that the generic drug will not have a poor effect on the person's condition.

- Ask if a lower dose can be prescribed without bad effects.

- To keep costs down, ask if a higher dose can be safely prescribed and the pill cut in half.

- Ask if you can buy a one-week supply of a new medication to see if the person can handle any possible side effects. Or ask if the physician has free samples to try.

> ### Tip
> **BUYING MEDICATIONS**
> Buying medications through mail order is often the cheapest way to buy. Ask if the insurance company has a mail-order program (see **Resources** *at the end of this chapter*).

Questions to Ask the Pharmacist

Some prescription drugs are not covered by health insurance, so shop around for the drug store with the lowest prices, and then stay with it. The pharmacist will come to know the care receiver's condition and can advise you about problems that might come up. Managed care plans are permitted to change doctor's orders by giving you a similar version that is cheaper. Do not try cutting drug costs without talking to your doctor about it first.

- Find out the highest allowable charge for a particular drug.

- Ask what over-the-counter drugs the pharmacist suggests for the person's condition (it may be necessary to take more of the drug if it is over-the-counter).

- Ask if the insurance company will pay for the drug the doctor prescribed.

- Ask if the doctor will be called to approve the switch to another drug.

- Find out what generic drug can be used instead of the prescription drug.

- Ask if the generic drug can cause side effects and when the doctor should be called about them.

- Ask if using more than one drug can cause unsafe drug interactions.

- Ask if the pharmacy's computer will alert the pharmacist about drug-interactions or side effects before the prescription is filled.

- Find out the risks of not taking the medicine.

- Find out the risks of not finishing the prescription.

- If you are caring for someone who will be taking several medications on his or her own, find a drug store that has easy-to-use packaging.

- Ask if the medicine can be put in a large easy-to-open container with a label in large print.

- Ask if an overdose of the medicine is dangerous.

- Ask if the medicine must be taken with a meal, with water or milk, etc.

- When the person needs many expensive drugs, find out if you can get a discount or work out a payment plan.

MEDICAL ALERT
An individual with a chronic medical condition who is mobile may want to wear a medical alert bracelet, or carry a card, that lists the medications she is currently taking.

MEDICAL RECORDS
To save costs, have all medical records and tests sent to the second doctor. Also, if possible, bring the important ones with you. Even the experts can disagree about the best treatment. The final decision is yours.

Alternative Treatments

A healthy lifestyle is encouraged by most medical providers. Use caution if you decide to try a different kind of treatment (known as complementary or alternative treatment). Look before you leap, and follow these commonsense guidelines:

- Be on guard against anyone who says to stop seeing a conventional (regular) doctor or to stop taking prescribed medicine.

- Look into the background of any treatment provider.

- Discuss the alternative or complementary therapy with your doctor.

- Figure out the costs of the treatments.

- Do not abandon conventional therapy.

- Keep a written account of the experience.

Mental Health Treatment

Strong emotions are a normal part of long-term illness. Counseling and support groups are a very helpful way of dealing with these feelings.

- For one who is depressed and needs therapy, ask the primary care doctor to give you the name of a therapist.

- Be aware that many people are embarrassed about mental health problems and may not want to seek care.

- For help determining a person's ability to make legal decisions, arrange for a geriatric psychiatrist's assessment.

Dental Care

Dental care is important for overall wellness. For low-cost dental programs, check with university dental schools or the local Area Agency on Aging.

- Tell the dentist all the medications the person is taking before starting dental treatment.

- Try to go to a dentist who is familiar with the person's disease.

- Find out how many visits will be needed each year.

- Ask if the office and dental chair are accessible, if that is needed.

- Ask about low-cost options to the treatment the dentist suggests.

- Ask if X rays are really necessary.

- Find out the cost of dentures, but don't trust prices that seem too good to be true. Cheap dentures may not fit correctly.

- When seeking another opinion, have all medical records and tests sent to the second dentist.

- Speak with the physician to determine if antibiotics are required prior to dental procedures.

Vision Care

Regular eye exams every two years by a specialist in eye disease (ophthalmologist) or someone who examines the eyes (optometrist) are necessary, especially after age 50. These exams can also spot or detect other serious diseases such as diabetes. Finding and treating disease early can prevent serious diseases from getting worse and leading to blindness.

- Tell the doctor of any medicines the person is taking.

- Tell the doctor if there is a family history of glaucoma.

- Get a yearly eye exam for a person with diabetes.

- Contact your state's Commission for the Blind for information on self-help organizations for those with low vision.

- Ask for help in finding products ("talking" watches, etc.) and aids that will help the person adjust to low vision.

 Danger signs to watch for are changes in the color or size of an object when one eye is covered or when straight poles appear bent or wavy. See an ophthalmologist (eye doctor) without delay.

How to Watch Out for Someone's Best Interests in the Hospital

A person in the hospital is at greater risk than others, so be ready to keep tabs on treatments, ask questions, and act as an advocate.

- If the Patients' Bill of Rights is not posted in a place where it can be seen, ask for a copy.

- Agree only to treatments that have been thoroughly explained.

- If something is not being done and you think it should be, ask why.

- Be friendly and show respect to hospital staff. They will probably respond better to you and to the person in your care. Bad feelings between family members and staff may cause the staff to avoid the person.

- Assist with the person's grooming and care.

- Speak up if you notice doctors or nurses examining anyone without first washing their hands.

- Check all bills and ask questions about anything that isn't clear to you.

 According to federal law, a hospital must release patients in a *safe manner* or else must keep them in the hospital. Letting a patient leave the hospital is not wise if the person has constant fever, infection or pain that cannot be controlled, confusion, disorientation (no sense of time or place), or is unable to take food and liquids by mouth. However, in some cases, it may be better for the person to be released because the noise and risk of catching other diseases may make it more difficult to recover. If you plan to appeal a discharge, understand the rules of Medicare, Medicaid, the HMO, or insurance plan.

When You Doubt the Time Is Right for Discharge

- Meet with the hospital's discharge planner.

- Ask if the hospital is following the usual policy for the condition.

- Explain any special reasons that make you think it is unwise to discharge the person.

- Ask if the hospital rules can be changed to cover this special case.

- Remember that anyone has the right to appeal a discharge.

- Get your doctor's help in the appeal, but understand that he or she may have different reasons for wanting to discharge the person.

Checklist Coming Home from the Hospital

✓ Assess the person's condition and needs.

✓ Understand the diagnosis (what is wrong) and prognosis (what will happen).

✓ Become part of the health care team (doctor, nurse, therapists) so you can learn how to provide care.

✓ Get complete written instructions from the doctor. If there is anything you don't understand, ASK QUESTIONS.

✓ Arrange follow-up care with the doctor.

✓ Develop a plan of care with the doctor. (📖 See **Setting Up a Plan of Care, Chapter 10**)

✓ Meet with the hospital's social worker or discharge planner to determine home care benefits and available services.

✓ Understand in-home assistance options. (See **Getting In-Home Help, Chapter 7**)

✓ Arrange for in-home help. The discharge planner can provide home health care agency names and arrange for these services.

✓ Arrange physical, occupational, and speech therapy as needed.

✓ Find out if medicine is provided by the hospital to take home. If not, you will have to have prescriptions filled before you take the person home.

✓ Prepare the home.

✓ Buy needed supplies; rent, borrow, or buy equipment such as wheelchairs, crutches, and walkers.

✓ Take home all personal items.

✓ Check with the hospital cashier for discharge payment requirements.

✓ Arrange transportation (an ambulance or van if your car will not do).

- State your doubts in a simple letter to the hospital's director or the health plan's medical director. (Rules vary from state to state.)

 Do not hesitate to call the hospital staff member who is responsible for patients' rights (typically called "ombudsman"). Most hospitals have an ombudsman department. This department is responsible for ensuring patients rights. They can be contacted regarding compliments and concerns about the hospital stay, and they help to resolve problems.

Case Management

Case management is an important resource for families living with chronic illness. It is easy to become stressed out with the demands of the disease and with the red tape of the health care and social services network. Case managers, who are typically nurses, need to have a basic understanding of the special needs of persons with chronic illness. Private insurance companies and Medicare supplement plans often provide case management services.

Case management skills are very helpful to families when there is a change in the person's physical state or in awareness and understanding. Should this happen, a case manager can take another look at the person's needs and at community supports. This may be necessary in the following instances:

- when the person loses the ability to process information and help is needed to identify issues and provide follow-up with a course of action

- when there is a change in the caregiver situation or support network that can easily become a crisis for the family as a whole

- when there are fewer financial resources and the family is no longer able to pay for the resources they need

- when safety issues arise that can put the ill person at greater risk

These issues and others require that case management continue as a long-term resource, so that the case manager can step in when needed to provide more support.

To learn more about case management or find a case manager in your area, contact:

- the National Association of Professional Geriatric Care Managers, Inc. at (520) 881-8008 or www.findacare manager.org

- your local Visiting Nurse Association

- Area Office on Aging

- hospital discharge planners

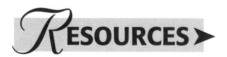

RESOURCES ▶

Go Ask Alice!
www.goaskalice.columbia.edu/about.html
Provides helpful information and lets you post health-related questions.

The Health Resource, Inc.
933 Faulkner Street
Conway, AR 72034
(800) 949-0090; (501) 329-5272; Fax (501) 329-9489
www.thehealthresource.com

Provides clients with personalized detailed reports on their specific medical conditions. These reports contain conventional and alternative treatments and information on current research, nutrition, self-help measures, specialists, and resource organizations. Reports on any non-cancer condition are $295, or $395 for complex issues, and contain 50 to 100 pages. Reports on any cancer condition are $395 and contain 150 to 200 pages. Shipping is additional.

http://hearthelp.com/
A great resource on heart topics and can help you locate a heart specialist in your area.

University of Washington
www.uwmedicine.org
A great storehouse of general health information on all topics.

Information About Eyesight

Lighthouse International
111 E. 59th Street
New York, NY 10022
(800) 829-0500
www.lighthouse.org

Lions Club International
300 W. 22nd Street
Oak Brook, IL 60523
www.lionsclub.org
(630) 571-5466

National Association for Visually Handicapped
22 West 21st Street, 6th floor
New York, NY 10010
(212) 889-3141
www.navh.org

National Federation of the Blind
1800 Johnson Street
Baltimore, MD 21230
(410) 659-9314
www.nfb.org

Medications

Together Rx Access® Card
A joint program by drug companies offering a free Prescription Savings Card for individuals and families who meet all four of the following requirements:

❐ *Not eligible for Medicare*

❐ *Have no public or private prescription drug coverage*

❐ *Household income equal to or less than:*

—*$30,000 for a single person*
—*$40,000 for a family of two*
—*$50,000 for a family of three*
—*$60,000 for a family of four*
—*$70,000 for a family of five*

❐ *Legal resident of the U.S. or Puerto Rico*

Call 1-800-250-2839 to start saving on your prescriptions. For the most current list of medicines and products, visit www. TogetherRxAccess.com

Publication

A *Family Caregiver's Guide to Hospital Discharge Planning*, a publication of the National Alliance for Caregiving and the United Hospital Fund of New York.
Available at www.caregiving.org

If you don't have access to the Internet, ask your local library to help you locate a Web site.

Getting In-Home Help

Getting In-Home Help

$\mathcal{G}$etting help with caregiving in the home involves the following options:

- **Using a home health care agency** (typical fee range: $50 to $150 per visit through a private agency)

- **Hiring someone privately** (typical fee range: $12 to $15 per hour; the cost of assistance is based on the category of professional or his or her experience)

- **Performing all caregiving duties with the assistance of family and friends.**

Use a Home Health Care Agency

Home Health Care Agencies are for-profit, nonprofit, or are run by the government. They provide personal care, skilled care, instructions for caregivers and the people in their care, and supervision. They usually provide certified nurse assistants (CNAs), sometimes called home health aides; registered nurses (RNs); licensed practical nurses (LPNs); physical therapists, occupational therapists, speech therapists, and social workers. (A doctor's order is required in order to get coverage for skilled-care nursing in the home.) These agencies help plan services and care that match the health, social, and financial needs of the client.

Definitions for Agencies

There are a number of terms to describe an agency's services and how it is able to do what it does. Study the terms carefully before looking into the agencies in your area.

Accredited—Services have been reviewed by a nonprofit organization interested in quality home health care.

Bonded—The agency has paid a fixed dollar amount in order to be bonded. In the event of a court action the bond pays the penalties. (Being bonded does not ensure good service.)

Certified—The agency has met the lowest federal standards for care and takes part in the Medicare program.

Certified Health Personnel—Those who work for the agency meet the standards of a licensing agency for the state.

Insurance Claims Honored—The agency will look into insurance benefits and will accept assignment of benefits (meaning the insurance company pays the agency directly).

Licensed—The agency has met the requirements to run its business (in those states that oversee home health care agencies).

Licensed Health Personnel—The personnel (staff) of the agency have passed the state licensing exam for that profession.

Screened—References have been checked; a criminal background check may or may not have been made.

How to Pay for Using an Agency

Paying for care from an agency ranges from Medicare to private pay to long-term-care insurance to state and county programs.

Medicare

To be eligible for the Medicare home-health benefit, a person must be basically unable to leave the house (homebound) and need skilled care.

- Medicare pays the full cost of medically necessary home health visits by a Medicare-approved home health agency.

- Medicare and most insurers will pay for skilled care (such as a registered nurse) that is not for maintenance.

- The person must be as unable to care for himself or herself as someone who would be in a nursing home.

NOTE State rules vary on who is eligible, so check with your area Medicare office for local rules.

State and County Personal Assistance Programs

- The person receiving services may need to be certified as eligible for a nursing home.

- Many programs require that the person be at a low-income level.

- Funding may come from Medicaid waivers and funding is sometimes not regular.

Private Pay

- If a person does not qualify for public funds, he or she must pay with long-term-care insurance or pay privately.

- Care management through Area Agencies on Aging may be free or offered on a sliding scale, based on a person's income.

What the Home Health Care Agency Will Do

- carry out an in-home visit

- look into insurance benefits and publicly funded benefits

- ask for an assignment of benefits (where payments are made by the insurer directly to the agency)

- ask you to sign a form to release medical information

- ask you to agree to and sign a service contract
- carry out an assessment (by the director of nurses) to determine the level of care required
- discuss the costs of suggested services
- come up with a plan of care that shows the person's diagnosis (what is wrong), functional limitations (what the person can and cannot do), medications, special diet, what services are provided by agency, advice for care, and list of equipment needed
- give you a written copy of the plan of care
- send a copy of the plan of care to the person's doctor
- select and send the right caregivers, only to the level of care needed, to the person's home
- adjust services to meet changing needs

Expect the Agency to:

- be an advocate, advisor, and service planner and to share information clearly with you
- give a full professional assessment
- get in touch with the care receiver's doctor as part of the assessment process
- have knowledge of long-term-care services and how to pay for them
- fill out the paperwork for publicly funded benefits
- show no bias or favor to service providers who may have contracts with the agency
- provide confidential treatment that will not be talked about with others

Checklist **Things to Do Before Selecting an Agency**

✓ Interview several agencies.

✓ Get references and CHECK THEM.

✓ Make a list of services you want and ask the agency what it will cost.

✓ Ask what the steps are in the care planning and management process and how long each will take.

✓ Find out how and when you can contact the care manager.

✓ Find out if the agency has a system for sending a substitute (stand-in) aide if the regular one doesn't show up.

✓ Ask if the agency will replace the aide if that aide and the person in care do not get along.

✓ Ask about the skills and ongoing training of personnel.

✓ Ask how they keep track of the quality of services.

✓ Ask for the services needed by the person in care, even if the insurance company is trying to hold down costs.

✓ Be aware that if a social service agency is providing the care services, they may limit you to only the services that they provide.

✓ Ask them to tell you about any referral-fee agreements they may have with nursing homes or other care facilities.

✓ Know what you have to do to lodge complaints against the agency with the state ombudsman or long-term-care office.

✓ Get in touch with the local/state Division for Aging Services to check for complaints against a particular agency.

- provide a written account of care when you ask for it

- have a proven track record of being honest, reliable, and trusted if the agency handles a person's money

Hire Someone Privately—A Personal Assistant

Even if you decide not to use an agency, a health care professional can help you decide how to prepare the home. They can give advice about needed supplies and where to purchase them and set up a care program. However, when you hire someone privately, you must assume payroll responsibility, complete required government forms (such as Social Security), decide on fringe benefits, track travel expenses, and provide a detailed list of tasks to be done.

WHEN YOU START CALLING FOR RESOURCES:

- Have information ready, such as what services will be needed and personal information, such as the age of the person, date of birth, social security number, etc.

- Have your questions written down and ready.

- Realize that to be eligible for some services there may be income, age, or geographic requirements.

- COMMUNICATE, COMMUNICATE, COMMUNICATE what you want and need!

Where to Find Help

- Yellow Pages under Nurses, Nursing Services, Social Service Organizations, Home Health Services, and Senior Services

- commercial agencies, which operate like temp employment agencies, screen applicants, and provide you with a list of candidates

- nonprofit agencies, such as the Visiting Nurse Association, which may charge a fee on a sliding scale (based on ability to pay)

- public health nursing through a county social service department (if you have no insurance or money)

- hospital discharge planner

- hospital-based home health agencies

- the school of nursing at a local community college

- college employment offices

- hospices (call the National Hospice Organization)

- nurses' registries

- Catholic Charities, Jewish Family Services, Lutheran Family Services and other faith-based groups

- the American Red Cross

- churches, synagogues, mosques

- a nearby nursing home employee who seeks part-time work

- an adult relative whom you would pay a fair hourly wage for services

Types of Health Care Professionals

Registered Nurse (RN)—has at least 2 years of school training and is licensed by the state Board of Nursing Examiners

Licensed Practical Nurse (LPN)—has finished a one- year course of study and is licensed by the state Board of Licensed Vocational Nurses

Certified Nurses Aide (CNA)—has finished 70 hours of classes and 50 hours of clinical practice in a nursing center setting; must pass a test and register with the State Board of Nursing

Home Health Aide—is screened on the basis of work experience; training and requirements differ from state to state

Someone who is taking classes or is in a training program that leads to one of the above professions might be able to help with care.

Tax Rules You Must Follow If You Hire Privately

- If you paid more than $1,400 in 2005 or $1,500 in 2007, you are required to pay Medicare and Social Security tax.

- You may use federal income tax return Form 1040 to pay the Social Security, Medicare, and Federal Unemployment (FUTA) taxes. Ask the Internal Revenue Service for the *Household Employer's Tax Guide*.

- For tax information, call the Social Security office. Look in the front of your phone book under State Government.

How to Screen a Personal Hire

- Check licenses, training, experience, and references.

- Be sure the person who is applying for hire has malpractice or liability insurance.

- Run a criminal background check and a driving record check (through a private investigator). Also, ask to see the person's insurance card.

- Find out if the person has a special skill (for example, working with care receivers who have heart failure).

- Decide whether the person is someone who can meet the emotional needs of the person in your care.

- Consider his or her personal habits.

- Find out if he is a smoker or nonsmoker.

Questions to Ask of the Applicant's References:

When someone is going to be hired, ask for the names of people who can tell you about this person's work and personal habits. Here are some questions you can ask:

- How long have you known this person?

- Did this person work for you?

- Is this person reliable, on time for work, patient, able to adjust as things change, able to be trusted, and polite?

- How does this person handle disagreements and emergencies?

- How well does this person follow directions, respond to requests, and take advice?

Perform All Caregiving Duties Yourself

If you decide to provide all the caregiving yourself, you can receive training at the following places:

- social service agencies

- hospitals

- community schools

- the American Red Cross

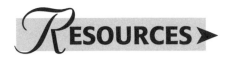

RESOURCES ➤

Family Caregiver Alliance
690 Market Street, Suite 600
San Francisco, CA 94104
(800) 445-8106; 415-434-3388 Fax: (415) 434-3508
www.caregiver.org
E-mail: info@caregiver.org
Resource center for caregivers of people with chronic disabling conditions. The Web site provides information on services and programs in education, research, and advocacy.

National Family Caregivers Association
10400 Connecticut Avenue, Suite 500
Kensington, MD 20895-3944
(800) 896-3650; (301) 942-6430
www.thefamilycaregiver.org
Email: info@thefamilycaregiver.org
The Association supports, empowers, educates, and speaks up for more than 50 million Americans who care for a chronically ill, aged, or disabled person.

Home Care Agencies/Hiring Help

The Center for Applied Gerontology, Council for Jewish Elderly
3003 W. Touhy Avenue
Chicago, IL 60645.
(773) 508-1000
E-mail: cag@cje.net
www.cje.net/professional/cag_orderform_2.pdf
Offers a 32-page pamphlet "Someone Who Cares: A Guide to Hiring an In-Home Caregiver." $9.95 plus $3.50 shipping and handling.

National Association for Home Care
228 Seventh Street, SE
Washington, DC 20003
(202) 547-7424
www.nahc.org
Provides referrals to state associations, which can refer callers to local agencies. Offers publications, including the free pamphlet "How to Choose a Home Care Agency: A Consumer's Guide." Information on finding help, interviewing, reference checking, training, being a good manager, maintaining a good working and personal relationship, problems that might arise and how best to solve them, service dogs, assistive technology, and tax responsibilities. Contains sample forms and letters.

Publications

Avoiding Attendants from Hell: A Practical Guide to Finding, Hiring and Keeping Personal Care Attendants by June Price, Science and Humanities Press

Managing Personal Assistants: A Consumer Guide, published by Paralyzed Veterans of America. To purchase a copy call (888) 860-7244, or download online at www.pva.org/cgi-bin/pvastore/products.cgi?id=2

If you don't have access to the Internet, ask your local library to help you locate a Web site.

Paying for Care

Paying for Care

You can look to many sources for help in paying for care. Some are public, while others are private or volunteer. The most common ways to pay for home care are as follows:

- *personal and family resources*

- *private insurance*

- *Medicare, Medicaid, Department of Veterans Affairs, and Title programs*

- *community-based services*

Assessment of Financial Resources

First, complete a personal financial resources assessment by doing the following steps:

- Look at current assets, where your income comes from, and insurance entitlements.

- Prepare a budget and figure out what your future income might be from all sources.

- Confirm the qualifications, retirement benefits, and Social Security status of the person in your care.

- Figure as closely as possible the expenses of professional care and equipment. Include any medical procedures likely to be needed.

- Check on the person's personal tax status and find out what care items and expenses are deductible.

- Find out if the person's health insurance or employer's workers' compensation policy has home health care benefits.

- Figure out how much money the person will need.

 Think about making the person in your care a "dependent" and thus be able to transfer medical expenses to a taxpayer who can make use of medical deductions.

Public Pay Programs

Medicare

Medicare is a federal health insurance program. It provides health care benefits to all Americans 65 and older and to those who have been determined to be "disabled" according to the Social Security Administration. After an individual has received Social Security Disability benefits for two years, they become eligible for Medicare benefits regardless of age. There are constant changes in Medicare policies, requirements, and forms. Therefore, it is always best to get the most current information on benefits by calling the Medicare Hotline (📖 See **Resources** at the end of this chapter) or your hospital's social worker.

Things That Affect Medicare Eligibility

Whether the Person Is Homebound—Medicare will pay for certain home health care services only if the person is confined to the home and requires part-time skilled (nursing) services or therapy. Medicare does not cover ongoing custodial (maintenance) care. "Confined to home" does not mean bedridden. It means that a person cannot leave home except for medical care and requires help to get there. (Brief absences from the home do not affect eligibility.)

In order for treatments, services, and supplies to be paid, they must be ordered by a doctor. They must also be provided by a home health agency certified by Medicare and the state health department.

Whether Care Is Intermittent (periodic)—In order to be covered, skilled services are required. Medicare is not designed to meet chronic ongoing needs that are considered "custodial" rather than "skilled."

Medicare Generally Pays for the Following:

- almost all costs of skilled care, such as doctors, nurses, and specialists

- various types of therapy—occupational, physical, speech-language

- home health services

- medical supplies and equipment

- personal care by home health aides (such as bathing, dressing, fixing meals, even light housekeeping and counseling) after discharge from a hospital or nursing home

Medicare Part D–Prescription Drug Plan

Beginning January 1, 2006, Medicare covers prescription drugs. There are two basic ways to sign up for this coverage. If you have traditional Medicare (Part A for hospital services and Part B for doctor and outpatient health care providers), you may sign up for a stand-alone Medicare Part D prescription drug plan. You can also choose a managed care plan under Medicare Advantage. These plans restrict you to only the doctors on the managed-care provider's list. They also have a prescription drug plan. All plans are from private companies that have been approved by Medicare (📖 See **Resources** at the end of this chapter).

Help is available to pay for copayments and premiums for those whose incomes are low enough to be eligible. A person must apply to the Social Security Administration for financial assistance.

> **NOTE** Phrases like "intermittent care," "skilled care," and "homebound" are not precisely defined. They are different from region to region, and the type and availability of coverage by Medicare may be different as well.

Services NOT covered by Medicare

Full-time nursing care at home, drugs, meals delivered to the home, homemaker chore services not related to care, and personal care services are usually not covered by Medicare.

> **NOTE** A caregiver who has power of attorney for a person on Medicare (the beneficiary) must send written permission to the person's Medicare Part B carrier. Send a letter with the person's name, number, signature, and a statement that the caregiver can act on behalf of the beneficiary. The form must list start and end dates.
>
> If there is a dispute about a repayment from Medicare, a review may be requested by filing a claim with the Medicare carrier.

Medicare Part B Insurance

Medicare Part B insurance costs between $96 and $238 per month (2008) and is based on yearly income. It offers extra benefits to basic Medicare coverage. It pays for tests, doctor's office visits, lab services, and home health care. A $135 deductible applies (2008). Medicare Parts A and B also cover some costs of organ transplantation.

Medicare Supplemental Insurance (Medigap)

To pay for benefits not covered by Medicare, this private health insurance option is available. It pays for noncovered services only—for example, hospital deductibles, doctor copayments, and eyeglasses—but does not cover long-term care services. Coverage depends on the plan you buy.

For anyone who has Medicare HMO coverage, Medigap insurance may not be necessary because those individuals only make a small copayment but do not pay a deductible for doctor's visits.

 It is illegal for an insurance company or agent to sell you a second Medigap policy unless you put in writing that you intend to end the Medigap policy you have. The federal toll-free telephone number for filing complaints is (800) 633-4227.

Medicaid

Medicaid pays for the medical care of low-income persons or those whose assets have been used up while paying for their own care. Eligibility depends on monthly income limits and personal assets. Coverage includes nursing facilities, assisted living, foster care, and certain types of home care. Each state runs its own Medicaid program, and so eligibility and coverage can vary. Some states have set up Medicaid Waiver programs, which pay for home and community-based services that would otherwise only be paid if one were in a nursing home.

Common Aspects of Medicaid

- Recipients must be financially and medically in need.

- For recipients who are terminally ill, benefits go on for as long as they are ill. However, care must be provided by an agency with hospice certification and Medicaid certification.

- Payments are made directly to providers of services.

- Long-term-care costs are paid for those not covered by insurance and for patients whose finances have run out.

- Payments to foster care homes and retirement communities are not covered (except in some cases by Medicaid waiver).

- Home health care services, medical supplies, and equipment are covered.

- Eligibility is based on a person's income and assets.

- People with disabilities who are eligible for state public assistance are eligible for Medicaid.

- People with disabilities eligible for Supplemental Social Security (SSI) are eligible for Medicaid.

- In many states, there are laws (called *spousal impoverishment laws*) that protect a portion of the estate and assets for the healthy spouse. These come into play after other monies have been "spent down" for the care of the ill spouse.

To find out what the benefits are, contact the local Social Security office, city or county public assistance office, or the Area Agency on Aging.

Services NOT covered by Medicaid

As a rule, Medicare, Medicaid, and private insurance do not cover many in-home services because they are not medical services. However, some community services may be called on to fill the gap for free or on a subsidized (public funding) basis. The following services usually are not covered but might be available locally free of charge:

- adult day care

- case management

- household chore services

- neighborhood and local meal services, such as Meals on Wheels

- consumer protection

- emergency response systems (which provide contact by phone or electronic device to police and rescue services)

- emergency assistance for food, clothing, or shelter

- friendly visitors (volunteers who stop by to write letters or run errands)

- services and equipment for those who have disabilities

- homemaker services

- legal and financial services

- respite care

- senior centers

- support groups (which will send materials if you write to them)

- telephone reassurance (volunteers who make calls to or receive calls from those who are elderly or living alone)

 The U.S. Congress and the Administration made major changes to Medicare and Medicaid, which will affect payment for long-term care. As these changes are put into effect, they are posted on the Web site of the Center for Medicare and Medicaid Services (CMS): www.cms.gov

Department of Veterans Affairs Benefits

Veterans generally qualify for health services in the home if a disability is service related. Even if a disability is not service related, other benefits may be available based on income qualifications. Some states have special programs only for veterans who live in that state. Some Veterans Hospitals have programs to deliver home health care services. Contact the nearest Veterans Affairs office or veterans group in your area.

Older Americans Act and Social Services Block Grant

Some agencies that provide support services get funding under this program. Services available may include the following:

- case management and assessment
- household chore services (minor household repairs, cleaning, yard work)
- companion services
- community meals
- home-delivered hot meals (Meals on Wheels) once or twice a day
- homemaker services
- transportation

Social Security Benefits

The Social Security Administration runs two federal disability retirement programs: Social Security Disability Insurance (SSDI) and Supplemental Security Income (SSI). SSDI is an insurance program that is funded by taxes from employees and employers. SSI is an assistance program for people with low incomes. The medical requirements and disability standards are the same.

Social Security considers a person disabled when he or she is unable to perform a paid job for which he or she is suited and the disability is expected to last for 12 months.

As a result of 2002 federal tax laws, people over 65 have no limits on the amount they can earn and still receive Social Security benefits. Call the Social Security Administration (1-800-772-1213) to get a report of your benefits record.

Understanding Social Security

- Retirement checks are loosely tied to how much a person paid into the system.

- Social Security provides the money for people who become disabled; once on disability for two years, the person would be eligible for Medicare benefits. If the person receiving Social Security dies, it also takes care of that person's spouse and children. The death benefit is $255.

- In 2007, Social Security typically pays $1,044 a month for the average retired worker.

- Social Security, personal savings, and employer pensions together provide financial support in old age.

NOTE Name the personal representative as co-renter of the safe deposit box if the person in your care does not have a spouse or close relative. This will make it easier to get into the safe deposit box after death.

Medicaid Guidelines

The cost of nursing home care is high and can easily wipe out a couple's savings even if only one person is in a nursing home.

Currently, Medicaid rules allow a person:

- to keep a home if he or she plans to return there or if it is lived in by a spouse or a disabled or minor child

- to have a maximum individual income (which varies state to state), including pension payments and Social Security

- to have a prepaid funeral fund of $1,500

- to have a bank account of no more than $2,000

General Points Regarding Asset Transfers

- Transfers must happen at least 60 months before applying to a nursing facility. (Transfers within 60 months may delay eligibility for Medicaid. Certain transfers from trusts can delay eligibility for up to 60 months.)

- A home can be transferred within 60 months if it is transferred to a spouse, a minor, or a disabled child.

- Transfers of assets to a child may be risky if the child will not be able or willing to help the parent if extra money is needed.

- A trust may be a better option because the money is still available for the parents' needs.

- If a person sets up a special-needs trust for himself, the assets must still be spent down to qualify for Medicaid payment for nursing home care.

- Among the penalties for people who transfer assets for less than fair market value to qualify for Medicaid is a $10,000 fine and up to a year in prison.

- The healthy spouse of a person who applies for Medicaid may retain some income and resources. Each case is assessed after the applicant becomes eligible for Medicaid.

- The most individual income a person can have and still get Medicaid varies from state to state. The rules can be tricky, so seek the advice of an attorney.

Employment Planning

Employment planning and retirement tips are very important. There are many issues to look into once the care receiver can no longer work. You will need to look at sick leave, short-term disability insurance, and the Family Medical Leave Act. When the person in your care decides to stop working, you will need to look into options for medical coverage. Applying for long-term disability benefits and Social Security can take a lot of time. You will need to find out what you can do while waiting for these new benefits.

You will also need to think about tapping into other sources of income once you decide to leave work: applying for Social Security, veterans benefits; the cash value of life insurance, long-term-care insurance; personal property, real estate, and mortgage insurance.

Health Maintenance Organizations (HMOs)

Health Maintenance Organizations are prepaid health insurance plans that give complete medical coverage for a fixed premium. Knowing whether an HMO is right for the person in your care requires careful study.

Types of HMOs

There are three types of HMOs:

IPA (Individual Practice Associations) Plans—A patient chooses a doctor from a primary care physician list.

POS (Point of Service) Plans—For an extra fee, a patient can visit a doctor outside of the network list.

Group Model HMOs—A patient must go to a clinic for treatment.

Remember, HMOs receive the same fees to treat a healthy person as a person with a chronic disease. For some patients with long-term or chronic illness, HMOs may not be a good choice. A patient who has a long-established relationship with a specialist who is not a member of the HMO's network list may not be able to continue to see that specialist.

 If a Medicare health plan is not meeting the needs of the person in your care, it is not difficult to switch to another plan or to a fee-for-service program.

How To Determine If an HMO Is Right for the Person in Your Care

- Ask if the doctor or specialist the person is now seeing is in the HMO network.

- Understand the person's medical needs—for special equipment, drugs, and help with activities. Determine if these needs are covered.

- Find out if the HMO is used to dealing with the illness the person has.

- Determine the specific services offered for this type of illness.

- Ask who decides what is medically necessary.

- Ask if there is a special Plan of Care for the illness.

- Ask if the person will get the *best* drugs for the condition or if generic substitutes will be offered.

- Ask how many people with this type of illness are under the plan in your area.

- Verify that the patient may see the specialists listed in the directory.

- Ask if the plan allows visits to specialists without a primary care doctor's referral.

- If a referral is required, find out how long it lasts and if a new referral is required for every visit.

- Ask what percentage of doctors on the list are board certified (have passed a special test given by the board of their specialty).

- Ask if the doctor has a financial incentive to do tests or to keep the patient from having tests or seeing a specialist.

- Ask if the plan covers visits to doctors outside the plan's referral list. (Out-of-network coverage may be limited to a certain dollar amount.)

- Ask how many doctors in the HMO specialize in geriatric care.

- If the person in your care must travel to a specific locale for extended stays, be sure the HMO allows visits to a different HMO there.

- Ask how the person will be charged if an emergency room visit is needed while traveling.

- Ask about the process for appealing a medical decision.

- Once you have decided on an HMO, get confirmation in writing regarding the items or services that are most important to the person in your care.

NOTE To find out how many patient complaints were registered against an HMO, call your state insurance commissioner in the phone book under State Government.

How to Appeal an HMO's Decision Regarding a Medical Procedure, Prescription, or Specialist Referral

When a treatment is denied, the goal is to reverse the denial as quickly as possible. Remember that the HMO can prolong a case in court, so the goal is to resolve the case without litigation.

- Call the HMO and ask for a copy of its formal appeals process. (Federal law requires HMOs to have such a process.)

- Make detailed notes of all conversations with the HMO; include the date and the staff person's name.

- Determine exactly why the HMO refused to cover the treatment.

- Ask the HMO clerk for an explanation; if the matter is not resolved, ask for the HMO medical director's explanation of denial of treatment.

- If you still feel the situation is not resolved, start a written appeal process.

- Ask the doctor for a written explanation why treatment is medically necessary (also ask the specialists you have visited for a letter of support).

- Save all bills related to the problem.

- For consumer advice or support for the appeal, call the state insurance department, state health department, advocacy group for the disease, or local Area Agency on Aging.

The clerk at the other end of the line is a person too, and being courteous always gets a better response than being viewed as irrational or disrespectful.

Community-Based Services

Many services are provided free by local or community groups. The groups are sometimes repaid by state, local, and federal governments, but often volunteers provide meals and social and health care services.

These services can sometimes make it possible for a person to stay at home and maintain independence.

Typical Services

Community-based services include the following:

Adult Day Care Centers, which provide services ranging from health assessment to social programs that help people with dementia or those at risk for nursing home placement.

Nutrition Sites, which serve meals in settings such as senior centers, housing projects, faith-based centers, and schools and sometimes provide transportation.

Meals on Wheels, which brings healthful food to the home.

Senior Centers, which offer a place to socialize and eat. (Often a hot meal at noontime on weekdays is the only one served.)

Transportation is offered by hospitals, nursing homes, local governments, and religious, civic, or other groups. Out-of-pocket costs vary and fees are set on a sliding scale based on ability to pay.

Do These Services Meet Your Needs?

For whatever need you have, there is most likely a program in your area. Here are some things to think about:

- Is the person the right age and income level to be eligible for the program?

- Is it necessary for the person to belong to a certain organization to be eligible?

- Is there a limit to how many times the person can use the services of the organization?

Where to Check

- local agencies (Catholic Charities, United Way, Jewish Family and Child Services, Lutheran Family Services)

- local churches, parishes, or congregations

- the government blue book pages under public service listings

- city or county public assistance offices

- rural areas (call the health agency in the county seat)

- personal doctor

- family services department

- hospital discharge planner or social worker

- insurance company

- local Area Agency on Aging

- previous or current employer (may have benefits)

- public health department

- Social Security office

- state insurance commission

- state or local ombudsman

The Area Agency on Aging can help find services in the community. It will know whether chore services, home-delivered meals, friendly visitors, and telephone reassurance are free of charge or are provided on a sliding scale.

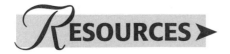

RESOURCES >

AARP
601 E. Street, NW
Washington, D.C. 20049
(800) 424-3410
www.aarp.org
Provides information on Medicare beneficiaries.

Centers for Medicare and Medicaid Services
7500 Security Boulevard
Baltimore, MD 21244-1850
(800) MEDICARE (633-4227) Medicare Hotline
www.cms.gov
www.medicare.gov
Federal agency that administers the Medicare and Medicaid programs, including hospice benefits.

National Association of Professional Geriatric Care Managers
1604 N. Country Club Road
Tucson, AZ 85716
(520) 881-8008
www.caremanager.org
Their Web site provides a free list of care managers in your state.

The National Council on the Aging
300 D Street SW, Suite 801
Washington, D.C. 20024
(202) 479-1200
www.ncoa.org
Provides a link to benefits (www.benefitscheckup.org) that helps seniors find state and federal benefits programs.

If you don't have access to the Internet, ask your local library to help you locate a Web site.

Planning for End-of-Life Care

Planning for End-of-Life Care

*B*esides deciding how to pay for long-term care, it is important to decide how future health care decisions will be made before things reach the crisis stage. These decisions should be recorded in legal documents for two reasons:

- *to make sure that a person's wishes are honored*

- *to make sure the family has enough information about those wishes in order to make life-and-death decisions*

The ability to plan for health care decisions depends on one's ability to:

- *understand the available treatment choices*

- *understand the results of those options*

- *make and communicate a thoughtful choice*

- *express values and goals*

Once these matters are understood, a range of legal documents can be drawn up to help ensure that the person's wishes will be carried out.

The following information is not intended as legal advice. We have presented a general summary of the rights of capable adults to make, or arrange for others to make, their health care decisions. Our summary does not contain all the technical details of laws in each state. Check what your state requires by law.

Directives for Health Care

There are two types of legal documents for indicating a person's wishes for advance directives if he or she is not able to make his or her own decisions. One type outlines the kind of medical attention the person wants, and the other names the person who will make sure these wishes are carried out. (The names of the documents may be different in your state.)

Living Will

A living will spells out a person's wishes about medical care in case he or she is physically unable to state those wishes. When drawing up a living will, it is important to consider a person's attitudes and desires regarding health care.

Health Care Proxy (Health Care Power of Attorney or Advance Directive)

This document allows a person to name someone as a personal representative (the health care proxy or representative) and gives that person the authority, or right, to carry out the person's wishes, as outlined in the living will.

Do Not Resuscitate Order (DNR)

A DNR or Do Not Resuscitate order is a written order from a doctor that CPR (cardiopulmonary resuscitation) should not be attempted if a person suffers respiratory or cardiac failure. This order can be obtained from the patient, or from someone entitled to make decisions on their behalf, such as a health care proxy (see above). This order can also be obtained on the basis of a physician's own initiative, usually when resuscitation would not change the ultimate outcome of a disease.

A DNR order can also have specific terms laid out in the order, such as no chest compression or intubation, but treatment for infections or other treatable conditions, intravenous feeding and fluids, pain management and comfort care to be continued.

For a DNR order to be valid there may be specific rules, such as the use of special forms and/or additional signatures, therefore check your state's policy.

Guardianship

Although not frequently needed, guardianship might be necessary if the person in your care becomes unable to make health care, personal or legal decisions. The guardian acts for an individual, usually referred to as the "ward." The guardian is appointed by the court to assume responsibility for the care and management of the person, the estate (or both) of the "incompetent" person. Obtaining guardianship is a legal process and in most states this is established through a probate court. To learn more about guardianship you can contact an attorney or the court system in your community.

Values History

This document explains a person's views on life and death and what he or she thinks is important. This can help the proxy or representative understand the person's wishes. It is a very helpful document because there is no way of knowing every medical situation that can possibly happen.

Why It Makes Sense to Prepare Directives

- They can be flexible and tailored to an individual's wishes.

- They apply to all health care situations.

- They may be given to anyone—a friend, relative, or spiritual advisor—to hold until needed.

- They are honored in the state where they were written and in most other states (check the state in question).

- They are not limited to issues of prolonging life but can also, for example, cover dental work and surgery.

- They can be created by filling out a standard form.

- Advance Health Care Directive forms are different from state to state and are available from most hospitals and nursing homes.

- They can be revoked (cancelled) at any time as long as the person is mentally able.

 It is important to have these legal and health documents for the person you are caring for. It is also important that you, the caregiver, have these documents drawn up for yourself.

Checklist **Do's and Don'ts in Planning Health Care**

✓ Do execute a new power of attorney or directive every few years to show that your wishes have not changed.

✓ Do use the proper form for your state.

✓ Do have the document drawn up by a lawyer so it follows the state rules.

✓ Do give a copy to the doctor, hospital, and any person holding power of attorney.

✓ Do ask the doctor and lawyer of the person in your care to review the document while that person is competent (mentally and physically able). Make sure they accept what is in it.

✓ Do keep a card with health care information in your wallet or that of the person in your care.

✓ Don't name the doctor as power of attorney.

✓ Do carry a copy of the document with you when you travel.

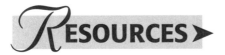

*R*ESOURCES ➤

AARP
(800) 424-3410
www.aarp.org
Can direct you to a hotline available in some states for brief legal advice by telephone to those 60 and older.

Administration on Aging
www.aoa.gov/legal/hotline.html
Web site lists legal hotlines for the states that have them for those 60 and older.

Caring Connections
(800) 658-8898
www.caringinfo.org
Distributes state-specific forms and explanatory guides for creating a living will.

The Equal Justice Network
www.equaljustice.org/hotline
A Web site sponsored by programs in the field offering legal advice over the telephone.

National Academy of Elder Law Attorneys
1604 N. Country Club Road
Tucson, AZ 85716
(520) 881-4005
www.naela.org
Provides a list of member lawyers in your area.

http://wings.buffalo.edu/faculty/research/bioethics/dnr-p.html This *Web site* is a helpful guide for patients and families looking into DNR orders.

Call your local **Social Security Administration, State Health Department, State Hospice Organization**, or call 1-800-633-4227 **Medicare Hotline** to learn about hospice benefits.

If you don't have access to the Internet, ask your local library to help you locate any Web site.

Part Two: Day by Day

Setting Up a Plan of Care

Setting Up a Plan of Care

A plan of care is a daily record of the care and treatment a person needs on a daily basis. The plan helps you and the person in your care with caregiving tasks.

When a person leaves a hospital, the discharge planner provides the caregiver with a copy of the doctor's orders and a brief set of instructions for care. The discharge planner also works with a home health care agency to send a nurse. The nurse will evaluate the patient's needs for equipment, personal care, help with shots or medication, etc. The nurse will also work with the entire health care team (including you as the caregiver, a physical therapist, and other specialists) to develop a detailed plan of care to be used on a daily basis.

The plan of care includes the following information:

- diagnosis (the nature of the disease)

- medications

- functional limitations (what the person can and cannot do)

- a list of equipment needed

- special diet

- detailed care instructions and comments

- services the home health care agency will provide, if using such an agency.

The information is presented in a certain order so that the process of care is repeated over and over until it becomes routine. When the plan is kept up to date, it provides a clear record of events that helps in solving problems and avoiding them.

With a plan, you don't have to rely on your memory. It also allows another person to take over respite care or take your place entirely without too much trouble.

Some of the things you may have to watch and record are

- skin color, warmth, and tone (dryness, firmness, etc.)

- breathing, temperature, pulse, and blood pressure (purchase a digital blood pressure cuff)

- circulation (dark red or blue spots on the legs or feet)

- fingernails and toenails (any unusual conditions)

- mobility (ability to move around) or ability to perform self-care (bathing, dressing, etc...)

- puffiness around the eyes and cheeks, swelling of the hands, abdomen, legs, ankles or feet.

- appetite (does the person in your care feel bloated or full quickly?)

- body posture (relaxed, twisted, or stiff)

- bowel and bladder function (unusual changes)

- daily weights

- amount of fluids and sodium consumed in a 24-hour period

Recording the Plan of Care

Use a loose-leaf notebook to record the plan of care. Put the doctor's instructions on the inside front cover (always keep the originals). Include in the notebook the types of forms that appear in the following pages of this chapter. These pages should be three-hole punched.

After using your plan of care for one week, make changes as needed and continue to do so as the person's needs change. Always do what works for you and the person in your care. Use notes, pictures, or anything else to describe your responsibilities. Also, use black ink, not pencil, to keep a permanent record.

Example Self-Care Log

Date	BP	Heart Rate	Weight	Fluid Intake	Sodium Intake	Symptoms
9/28	84/43	82	143 pounds	59 ounces	1650 mg	
9/29	72/40	80	146 pounds	70 ounces	2000 mg	Felt dizzy when getting up. Feel swollen today and weight is up 3 pounds overnight. Will call MD.

Recording and Managing Medications

Always be sure that the person in your care takes the medication exactly as prescribed. Keep an accurate list of these medications and when they should be taken.

Never make any changes to these medications without talking to the doctor or specialist first. However, because everyone's treatment needs are different, the specialist may want to try changing the amount or timing of drugs, within certain limits. If you are worried or have any questions, don't be afraid to ask your doctor or pharmacist for advice.

People who have serious health problems often take a large number of medications at many different times of the day. It is essential to have a careful system for keeping track of medications:

- when medications should be given

- how they should be given

- when they were actually given

The following sample of a weekly medication schedule is a good model to follow. Be sure to fill in the times when (am and pm) medications actually were given, and have each caregiver initial them.

Weekly Medication Schedule (Sample Form)

Medication	Date/Time/Initials						
Name, dose, frequency, with or without food	Sat.	Sun.	Mon.	Tues.	Wed.	Thurs.	Fri.
Example							
Coumadin 2 mg *1x daily a.m. with food*							
Folic acid 400 mg *1x daily a.m.*							
Vitamin/mineral capsule *1x daily, with food* • *Noon*							
Artificial tears *2x daily* • *8 a.m.* • *bedtime*							

As you finish your own schedule, be sure to record information from the label of each prescription, including:

- days of the week when each medicine must be taken

- number of times per day

- time of day

- whether the medicine is to be taken with or without food

- how much water should be taken with the medicine

Also make a note to yourself about any warnings (for example, "Don't take this medicine with alcohol") and possible side effects (dizziness, confusion, headache, etc.).

> **NOTE** Labels may contain the following abbreviations that you should be aware of:
>
> **HS**—hour of sleep (medication time)
> **BID**—give the medicine 2 times per day (approximately 8 am and 8 pm)
> **TID**—give the medicine 3 times per day (approximately 9 am, 1 pm, 6 pm)
> **QID**—give the medicine 4 times per day (approximately 9 am, 1 pm, 5 pm, 9 pm)

Other Cautions

- Never crush pills without talking to the doctor or pharmacist first. If the person in your care has trouble swallowing medication, ask the doctor if there is another way it can be taken. (📖 See *Using the Health Care Team Effectively,* **Chapter 6**)

- If the person in your care will take the medicine without your help, ask the pharmacist to use easy-open caps on prescription bottles.

- Do not store medicine that will be taken internally (swallowed) in the same cabinet with medicine that will be used externally (lotions, salves, creams, etc.).

- Keep a magnifying glass near the medicine cabinet for reading small print.

- Store most medicine in a cool, dry place—usually not the bathroom.

- Remove the cotton from each bottle so that moisture is not drawn in.

- Check with your pharmacist about disposal options for expired medications in your area. Dispose of needles in the sharp containers and return to the appropriate agency (local pharmacy, doctor's office, local hospital etc.).

Tip

EMERGENCY PREPAREDNESS

Let the local fire station and ambulance company know that a person with disabilities lives at your address. They will have the information on hand and can respond quickly.

Emergency Information

Have this information posted near telephones or on the refrigerator, where it can be used by anyone in the household in case of emergency.

Personal Information

Name _____ Date of Birth _____

Address _____

Phone _____

SS # _____ Supplemental Insurance # _____

Medicaid # _____ Medicare # _____

Current Medications: _____

_____

Exact Location of Do Not Resuscitate Order: _____

Emergency Numbers

Fire _____ Police _____

Ambulance _____ Hospital _____

Doctor _____

Drugstore _____ Open Till _____ Delivers _____

Family Caregiver Work Number _____

Alternate Caregiver _____

Home Health Care Agency _____

Medicare Toll Free Number _____

Insurance _____

Medical Equipment Company _____

Poison Control _____

Friend _____

_____

Neighbor _____ Relative _____

Clergy/Rabbi _____

Transport Number _____ Meals-on-Wheels _____

Shopping Assistance _____

_____

Directions for Driving to the House _____

_____

_____

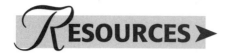

RESOURCES

Elder Health Program
Peter Lamy Center on Drug Therapy and Aging
University of Maryland at Baltimore
School of Pharmacy
506 West Fayette Street, Room 106
Baltimore, MD 21201
(410) 706-7434; Fax (410) 706-1488
www.pharmacy.umaryland.edu/lamy
Provides free information about older people and medications.

General Caregiving Books
Always on Call: When Illness Turns Families into Caregivers, by Carol Levine (Ed.).
New York United Hospital Fund, 2000.

The Complete Eldercare Planner, by Joy Loverde.
Three Rivers Press, 2000.

Taking Care of Aging Family Members, by Wendy Lustbader, New York. Free Press, 1994.

If you don't have home access to the Internet, ask your local library to help you locate any Web site.

How to Avoid Caregiver Burnout

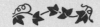

How to Avoid Caregiver Burnout

*P*roviding emotional support and the physical care for an ill person can be very satisfying and rewarding. But it is an enormous responsibility as well, and people can feel very stressed. In addition to providing care for the patient, the caregiver may still be trying to work outside of the home, take care of other family members, and manage extra home responsibilities. Balancing all of these jobs may lead you to feel overwhelmed, angry, and guilty.

One of the biggest mistakes caregivers make is thinking that they can—and should—do everything by themselves. The best way to avoid burnout is to have the practical and emotional support of other people. Sharing concerns with others can relieve stress, give you practical assistance, and help you find solutions to care and home situations. It can truly lighten your load.

Negative Emotions That May Arise in You

The challenges of the caregiver role may sometimes make you feel bad about yourself. If you are a perfectionist, you'll never do it perfectly. If you're angry, you'll find plenty of excuses to be mad. If you have feelings of inadequacy, they'll definitely come up. Impatience, depression, hostility—if these emotions challenged you before, they're sure to arise in this situation.

Guilt Is Crippling

Opportunities for guilt can come up often in caregiving. Even if you are doing it perfectly, you can easily convince yourself that you're not doing enough. To combat this tendency, *at least once a day, every day*, remind yourself:

- about how you are helping the person in your care
- when you don't do things perfectly, you are doing them with love
- you have grown in skill and compassion

Depression Is Dangerous

Just as depression endangers the recovery of the person in your care, it also endangers *your* health and well-being. Depression increases your risk in every major disease category, particularly cardiovascular disease. Studies have shown that a high percentage of caregivers develop symptoms of depression. However, there are ways you can reduce and prevent the chances of becoming depressed, as you will read about later in this chapter.

Symptoms of Depression

Here are the symptoms:

- persistent sad, anxious or "empty" mood
- feelings of hopelessness, pessimism
- feelings of guilt, worthlessness, helplessness
- loss of interest or pleasure in hobbies and activities that were once enjoyed, including sex
- decreased energy, fatigue, being "slowed down"
- difficulty concentrating, remembering, making decisions
- insomnia, early-morning awakening, middle of the night awakening or oversleeping
- appetite and/or weight changes
- thoughts of death or suicide, or suicidal attempts
- restlessness, irritability

If you have five or more of these symptoms for longer than two weeks, depression may be the cause. Talk to a physician, psychiatrist, psychologist, or clinical social worker about treatment options. The most effective treatment combines medication with talking therapy.

• Claim time for yourself and make sure you use it; otherwise, you will burn out and the person in your care will suffer.

• Make and keep doctor's appointments for yourself; otherwise, when you get sick, everyone will suffer.

• Join a caregiver support group. This website: www.chfpatients.com/heartforum.htm offers information about support group meetings. It also offers a forum or question section. It may help you and the person in your care feel less isolated.

• Take advantage of respite care opportunities, otherwise, when you break down the person in your care will suffer.

Anger

It is easy to feel victimized in this situation; you are caught up in someone else's illness. The natural response is anger. Unfortunately, that is not a helpful response. Unleashing anger on the person in your care never helps.

On the other hand, it is not good for you to stuff those feelings. There are definite consequences to your health and well-being. Try these outlets:

• Caregiver support groups provide a place where you can vent feelings. Everyone there understands; no one will make you feel guilty. Members will often offer effective, real-world solutions. Scientific evidence indicates caregivers who participate in support groups are better able to deal with the situation.

- Make an appointment with a therapist or family counselor or clergyperson. If possible, make two appointments: one for you alone and one for you and the person in your care.

- Keep a journal of your feelings.

- Take some time every day just for you—at least 15 minutes when you take a time out for yourself. Create a respite zone, which we will talk more about at the end of this chapter.

- Remember, people who have lost control may try to regain it by controlling what they can, which may be their caregivers.

- Separate the person from the condition. The illness, not the person in your care, is responsible for the difficulties and challenges that you both are facing. Don't blame the care receiver for the situation you are in.

- Set and enforce limits on how many non-essential needs you will fill per hour, such as pouring water or changing channels. Non-emergency care does not have to be handled immediately.

Tip

Sometimes it is necessary to tell the person in your care how you are feeling, but it is important not to accuse him personally. Saying "You make me feel angry" may worsen the situation. Instead say, "Just as I am trying to understand what you are going through, please try to understand what I am going through with you."

Emotional Burdens

You may think you are the only one to face these problems, but you are not alone. Every caregiver faces—

- the need to hide his or her grief
- fear of the future
- worries about money
- having less ability to solve problems

Dependency and Isolation

Fears of dependency and loneliness, or isolation, are common in families of those who are ill. The person needing care can become more and more dependent on the one who is providing it. At the same time, the caregiver needs others for respite and support. Many caregivers are ashamed about needing help, so they don't ask for it. Those caregivers who are able to develop personal and social support have a greater sense of well-being.

NOTE Men who are caregivers face special problems. Often they are not used to doing daily chores around the house. They also lose the emotional support of the spouse who is ill and must now be her support. It is especially important for men to seek out a support system. One study showed that when male caregivers approached and organized home tasks in the same way they did their work outside of the home, they felt less stress.

Knowing When to Seek Help

"Why doesn't anyone ask how I am doing?" It is easy to feel invisible, as if no one can see you. Everyone's attention is on the person with the illness, and they don't seem to understand what the caregiver is going through. Many caregivers say that nobody even asks how they're doing. Mental health experts say it's not wise to let feelings of neglect build up. Caregivers need to speak up and tell other people what they need and how they feel.

Support groups, religious or spiritual advisors, or mental health counselors can teach you new and positive ways to express your own need for help.

Seek out professional help when you:

• are using more alcohol than usual to relax

• are using too many prescription medications

• have physical symptoms such as skin rashes, backaches, or a cold or flu that won't go away

• are unable to think clearly or focus

• feel tired and don't want to do anything

• feel keyed up, on edge and irritable

• feel sad much of the time and find yourself crying more than normal for you

• feel intense fear and anxiety

• feel worthless and guilty

• are depressed for two weeks or more

• are having thoughts of suicide

• have become or are thinking about becoming physically violent toward the person you are caring for

When Hostility Builds to the Breaking Point

Anger is a common emotion for caregivers and for the person being cared for. The situation feels—and is—unfair. Both may say hurtful words during a difficult task. Someone may slam a door during a disagreement. Shouting sometimes replaces conversation. Anger and frustration must be addressed and healthy outlets found as a way to let off steam. If they are not, angry situations can become physically

Checklist Dealing with Physical and Emotional Burdens

✓ Do not allow the person in your care to take unfair advantage of you by being overly demanding.

✓ Live one day at a time.

✓ List priorities, decide what to leave undone, and think of ways to make the work easier.

✓ When doing a long, boring care task, use the time to relax or listen to music.

✓ Find time for regular exercise to increase your energy (even if you only stretch in place).

✓ Take several short rests in order to get enough sleep.

✓ Set aside time for prayer or reflection.

✓ Practice deep breathing and learn to meditate to empty your mind of all troubles.

✓ Realize your own limitations and accept them.

✓ Make sure your goals are realistic—you may be unable to do everything you could do before.

✓ Keep your eating habits balanced—do not fall into a toast-and-tea habit.

✓ Take time for yourself.

✓ Treat yourself to a massage.

✓ Keep up with outside friends and activities.

✓ Spread the word that you would welcome some help, and allow friends to help with respite care. It can be hard to ask for help, but you can't do the whole job alone.

✓ Delegate (assign) jobs to others. Keep a list of tasks you need to have done and assign specific ones when people offer to help.

✓ Share your concerns with a friend.

✓ Join a support group, or start one (to share ideas and resources).

✓ Use respite care when needed.

✓ Express yourself openly and honestly with people you feel should be doing more to help.

✓ When you visit your own doctor, be sure to explain your caregiving responsibilities, not just your symptoms.

✓ Allow yourself to feel your emotions without guilt. They are natural and very human.

✓ Unload your anger and frustration by writing it down.

✓ Allow yourself to cry and sob.

✓ Know that you are providing a very important service to the person in your care.

or emotionally abusive. (📖 See **Abuse section**, page 202). You can control your emotions by letting go of anger and frustration in a safe way.

- Take a walk to cool down.

- Write your thoughts in a journal.

- Go to a private corner and take out your anger on a big pillow.

- Make time for yourself each day. Do something just for you, even if it is for only 15 minutes. Break the cycle of helping others for a brief time; instead help yourself.

Where to Find Professional Help or Support Groups

- the community pages of the phone directory
- the local county medical society, which can provide a list of counselors, psychologists, and psychiatrists
- religious service agencies
- community health clinics
- religious and spiritual advisors
- United Way's "First Call for Help"
- a hospital's social service department
- a newspaper calendar listing of support group meetings
- parish nurses
- Area Agency on Aging

Ask for help from a counselor who is familiar with the needs of caregivers.

Self-Care for Caregivers

If you don't take care of yourself, then you won't finish the caregiving race, and the care receiver will suffer. Part of your responsibility to the person in your care is to take care of yourself.

Here's a thought to keep in mind: In the safety talk before every flight, the stewardess tells parents to put the oxygen mask on themselves first and then the child. Why? Because if the parent passes out, the child's safety is at risk.

Exercise

Even moderate exercise is beneficial because it breaks the cycle of being sedentary. And being sedentary is a risk factor for all major diseases.

Walking is easy, and if you can't walk for 30–40 minutes at a stretch, several 5–10 minute periods are enough. Exercise improves mood and physical well-being and can be an opportunity to socialize. Find a way to make it part of your day. If you feel that you cannot leave your home, there are exercise DVDs and videos that will allow you to implement an exercise routine in your home, while still being alert to the person in your care. Remember, you want to allow *at least* 15 minutes for yourself each day.

If you can't join a gym, investigate the YMCA. Some larger churches often have low- or no-cost exercise classes.

Eat Right

Nutrition is critical to your well-being. Learn to read labels and avoid foods with high fat content. Monitor your portion size; for example, a proper serving of meat is about the size of a deck of playing cards.

The person in your care will almost certainly be given a dietary prescription. In cooking heart-healthy for him, you will benefit yourself and the rest of your family. (📖 See **Diet, Nutrition, and Exercise,** page 209).

 Tip

Calorie-dense foods pack a lot of calories in a small package—think chocolate. For example, 8 oz of broccoli is 65 calories; 8 oz of chocolate chip cookies is 1,070 calories. Fresh fruits and vegetables will typically have many fewer calories than processed foods. Canned fruit often has added sugar; canned vegetables generally have added salt.

Tip

Most people need to eat more fruit—9 servings a day. To help you meet that goal, keep a bowl of apples, oranges, pears, bananas, and seasonal fruits on a kitchen counter and nibble on the fruit throughout the day.

Tip

For reliable and easy-to-understand information on nutrition; changing your diet; easy-to-follow eating plans; and quick, tasty, and healthy recipes, go to www.AmericanHeart.org. It is a free, one-stop shop for heart-healthy nutrition.

Take Care of the Caregiver

Being a caregiver can be the most rewarding job of your life, but also the hardest and most demanding. It does not mean you have failed when you find you can't provide 100 percent of the care yourself. It means you are wise and respect yourself when you ask for help.

Many caregivers neglect their own physical health. They ignore what is ailing them and don't take steps to avoid getting sick, such as exercising, eating a proper diet, and getting regular medical examinations.

Many caregivers do not get enough sleep at night. If sleep is regularly broken up because the person in your care needs help during the night, talk about the problems with a health care professional.

The person in your care needs a healthy caregiver. Both partners need uninterrupted sleep.

Meditation

Your journey as a caregiver will be more satisfying and less stressful if you take up a practice of daily meditation. Think of meditation as sitting still doing nothing. Here are seven easy steps:

1. Sit so your back is straight, either on a chair or a big, firm pillow.

2. As you inhale, tense your whole body—arms, legs, buttocks, fists, scrunch your face.

3. Hold 2–3 seconds.

4. Exhale and relax (repeat twice).

5. Take a deep breath, let your belly expand.

6. Exhale and relax (repeat twice).

7. Breathe normally and observe your thoughts for five minutes.

Most people fail at meditation because they think meditation means clearing your mind of thoughts. Instead of emptying your mind of thoughts, observe them. There are no "right" thoughts to think. Don't focus on any of your thoughts and don't fight with any of them. An easy way to do that is to label each one as it bubbles up—sad thought, happy thought, angry thought, depressed thought, to-do list thought—and let it go and then label the next one that appears.

 A kitchen timer will alert you to five minutes.

 It is not important how long you sit with your eyes closed and observe your thoughts—5 minutes will do, especially to start. What makes meditation effective at reducing stress is the *practice* of meditation, doing it every day. **You can do it before the person in your care wakes up or after she goes to bed or is taking a nap. It's only 5 or 10 minutes, but the cumulative effect over just a few weeks is noticeable.**

Plan for the Long Term: Winning the Caregiving Race

Most people jump into caregiving as if it were a sprint. They think they can and must do everything themselves. You may be able to do that for a few weeks or even months, but the average caregiver spends more than four years in that role—no one can sprint for that long. Because of advances in health care, people are surviving longer with chronic medical conditions. They may also be sent home from the hospital with more care needs. This only points out two more reasons why you, as the caregiver, should pace and care for yourself as well.

Instead of a sprint, treat caregiving as a marathon—for which you have not trained—and pace yourself accordingly from the start. Find effective ways to share or get help from others.

Respite Time

Every caregiver needs respite time if she is to last. It may be hard to think of yourself and your needs at this time, but if you don't, your life will be consumed by your duties and you will burn out. Respite (a temporary break from responsibility) is not a luxury, it is a necessity.

Your care receiver's level of disability determines whether he or she can be left alone and for how long. Care options include—

- asking a family member or friend to stay with your care receiver for an hour or two

- taking him or her to adult daycare (if ambulatory)

- employing a professional sitter or health care aide for a few hours a week or month

- hiring a college student (if skilled care is not needed) to stay with your care receiver

- enrolling the person in your care in a support group

Check with your local Area Agency on Aging for respite-care programs in your area. Larger churches often have outreach programs that include respite care.

However you are able to arrange for some help—and it will take some effort on your part, it won't happen by itself—commit to taking some time at least once a week to do something for yourself, preferably outside of the house.

NOTE To make this happen you will have to defend this time because other people and tasks can easily become a priority. If you do not defend your respite time, you will not get it or the renewal it generates. Remember, caregiving is a marathon, not a sprint—respite time helps you finish the race.

Respite Zone

A respite zone is an area within your home set aside just for you, the caregiver. The idea is that this is your space. It can be your bedroom, the spare room, an office, or even a bench outside in the garden or on a porch. This is a place for you to take a break while the person in your care rests or is taken care of by someone else.

In creating your respite zone,

- Keep in mind what you want to do there. Reading? Painting? Writing? Gardening? Bubble bath?

- Identify the time you will use it—during nap time, when someone spells you? If you can only get a break at night after the person in your care is in bed, gardening probably won't do.

- Identify free space in your home—porches are good candidates, a spare room is perfect, maybe a corner of your bedroom. A screen can give you privacy if you can't close the door.

- Modify the space according to your needs—a reading chair with a lamp or a stereo headset. Keep whatever is necessary for your respite activity.

Your respite zone should be your creation alone. The goal is to give you a place of your own where you can find enjoyment in your own home and life. If searching the Internet is fun for you, your zone will be different from someone who wants to take a bubble bath and listen to soft music. Creative projects such as painting, sewing, writing, baking, gardening, and photography are excellent ways to absorb your attention and take your mind off your responsibilities.

Your respite zone should be just for you. You need to feel secure that your things are safe and will not be disturbed or discarded. It is important for your care receiver to understand that this space is yours.

Tip

It is not selfish to set aside space and time for yourself, because if you fail to give yourself space, time, and the opportunity to be with your own thoughts, your caregiving journey will be harder on you than it has to be.

Taking care of a debilitated (weakened) family member or friend who may not recover completely can be an all-consuming job. However, if you allow it to consume all of you because you do not demand some time and space for yourself, what will happen to the person in your care when you collapse?

Respite care is not a luxury. It is necessary for the well-being of the person in your care and for you.

Changes in Attitude Relieve Stress

Here are some suggestions to help reduce your stress level:

- Learn to say no. Good boundaries improve relationships.

- Control your attitude: Don't dwell on what you lack or what you can't change.

- Appreciate what you have and can do.

- Go on a TV diet. Find simple ways to have fun: Play a board game, organize family photos, listen to music you enjoy, read the biography of an inspiring person.

- Learn a time-management tool, like making a to-do list (specifically include items that you enjoy).

- Knowledge is empowering; get information about heart failure. Encourage the person in your care to control what they can about their condition, such as diet, taking medications and keeping doctor's appointments.

- Limit coffee and caffeine.

- Find a support system and nurture it.

- Share your feelings with someone who wants to listen. Talking with a close and understanding friend is good medicine for anyone.

- Keep a gratitude journal—record three new things you are grateful for every day.

- Memorize an inspiring poem.

> **NOTE** The #1 thing you can do to improve your situation is to acknowledge your role. A survey of family caregivers by the National Family Caregivers Association showed that spouse caregivers often refuse to accept that caregiving is a separate role to the role of spouse. The survey found that shifting this attitude—accepting that caregiving is a separate role—had a profound impact on their situation.

The job of long-term caregiving is too big for one person—no matter how much love the caregiver has for the person in her care. Ask for and accept help from as many sources as you can find.

Outside Activities

Successful caregivers don't give up their own enjoyable activities. Many organizations have respite care programs to provide a break for caregivers. Other family members are often willing—even pleased—to spend time with the person. It may be possible to have respite care on a regular basis. Keep a list of the people you can ask for help once in a while.

If your friends want to know how they can help ease your burden, ask them to:

- telephone and be a good listener as you may voice strong feelings

- offer words of appreciation for your efforts

- share a meal

- help you find useful information about community resources

- show genuine interest

- stop by or send cards, letters, pictures, or humorous newspaper clippings

- share the workload

- help hire a relief caregiver

It helps to remember the saying, "Grant me the serenity to accept the things I cannot change, the courage to change the things I can, and the wisdom to know the difference."

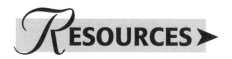

RESOURCES

Caregiver Survival Resources
www.caregiver911.com
A comprehensive list linking caregiving information and services for general issues and specific chronic illnesses.

Caring.com

www.caring.com

Help with concerns about caregiving and advice from trusted experts in medicine, legal matters, finances, housing, and family issues, as well as community support from caregivers like you.

Center for Family Caregivers/Tad Publishing Co.

www.caregiving.com or www.familycaregivers.org

Develops and distributes educational materials on care-giving, including a newsletter. Caregiving informational kits are $5 each; please specify new, seasoned, and transitioning caregiver when requesting a kit.

Eldercare Locator

(800) 677-1116

www.eldercare.gov

Provides information about local support resources offering services to the elderly.

Lotsa Helping Hands

www.lotsahelpinghands.com

Provides a free-of-charge Web service that allows family, friends, neighbors, and colleagues to assist more easily with daily meals, rides, shopping, baby-sitting, and errands that may become a burden during times of medical crisis.

National Alliance for Caregiving

4720 Montgomery Lane, 5th Floor

Bethesda, MD 20184

www.caregiving.org

The Alliance is a non-profit coalition of national organizations focusing on issues of family caregiving.

National Family Caregivers Association
10400 Connecticut Avenue, Suite 500
Kensington, MD 20895
(800) 896-3650
info@thefamilycaregiver.org
www.thefamilycaregiver.org
Free member benefits include Take Care!, a quarterly newsletter;
The Resourceful Caregiver, a useful guide to resources; a support
hotline and online chat room.

The Beat Goes On
Heart Failure Support Group
www.chfpatients.com/heartforum.htm

Today's Caregiver Magazine
6365 Taft Street, Suite 3003
Hollywood, FL 33024
(800) 829-2734
www.caregiver.com/magazine
Bimonthly magazine dedicated to caregivers.

Well Spouse Association
63 West Main Street, Suite H
Freehold, NJ 07728
(800) 838-0879
info@wellspouse.org
www.wellspouse.org
Publishes Mainstay, a bimonthly newsletter and provides net-
working/local support groups.

Check with your local church or health facility to see
if they sponsor **Share the Care** teams.

Publications

A Caregiver's Survival Guide: How to Stay Healthy When Your Loved One Is Sick, by Kay Marshall Strom. Intervarsity Press, 2000.

Care for the Family Caregiver: A Place to Start, a report prepared by HIP Health Plan of New York and National Alliance for Caregiving. Available at www.caregiving.org

Caring for Yourself While Caring for Others: A Caregiver's Survival and Renewal Guide, by Lawrence M. Brammer. Vantage Press, 1999.

Caring for Yourself While Caring for Your Aging Parents: How to Help, How to Survive, by Claire Berman. Henry Holt, 1996.

Helping Yourself Help Others: A Book for Caregivers, by Rosalynn Carter, with Susan Golant. Random House/Time Books, 1995.
(800) 733-3000
Plenty of basic information for caregivers.

A Family Caregiver Speaks Up, by Suzanne Geffen Mintz. Capital Books, 2007.

Mainstay: For the Well Spouse of the Chronically Ill, by Maggie Strong.

Positive Caregiver Attitudes by James Sherman, PhD.

The Emotional Survival Guide for Caregivers by Barry J. Jacobs, PsyD. The Guilford Press., 2006.

The Fearless Caregiver: How to Get the Best Care From Your Loved One and Still Have a Life of Your Own, by Gary Bang. Capital Books, 2001.

If you don't have home access to the Internet, ask your local library to help you locate any Web site.

Activities of Daily Living

Activities of Daily Living

Personal Hygiene

As a caregiver, you may find that some of your time each day will be devoted to assisting the person in your care with personal hygiene. This includes bathing, shampooing, oral or mouth care, shaving, and foot care. Even though the person in your care needs assistance, encourage them to help you and to do whatever they can for themselves. They will likely feel less dependent and you may feel less burdened. If you have the assistance of a home health aide, they may help with the bath.

The Bed Bath

Bed baths are needed by people who are confined to bed. Baths clean, stimulate, and increase blood flow (circulation) in the skin. However, they can also dry the skin and in some instances cause chapping. Thus, you must decide how often a bed bath is needed. Your decision must be based on the situation of the person in your care. For example, if urinary incontinence (leakage), bowel problems, and heavy perspiration are present, a daily bath may be in order. If not, bathing 2 to 3 times a week might be enough. At bath time, inspect the whole body for pressure sores, swelling, rashes, moles, and other unusual conditions. If baths are given often and the skin is dry, use soap and water one time and lotion and water the next. Cornstarch and powder can cause skin problems in some people. Ask the nurse on your health care team for advice.

SKIN CARE

It is easier to prevent chapping than to heal it, so apply lotion often.

To avoid spreading germs, always wash your own hands before and after giving a bath. At each step, tell the person what you are about to do and ask for his help if he is able.

1. Make sure the room is a comfortable temperature and not too warm.

2. Gather supplies—disposable gloves, mild soap, washcloth, washbasin, lotion, comb, electric razor, shampoo—and clean clothes.

3. Use good body mechanics (position)—keep your feet separated, stand firmly, bend your knees, and keep your back in a neutral position.

4. Offer the bedpan or urinal.

5. If you have a hospital bed, raise the bed to its highest level and bring the head of the bed to an upright position.

6. Help with oral hygiene—brushing the teeth or cleansing the mouth.

7. Test the temperature of the water in the basin with your hand.

8. Remove the person's clothes, the blanket, and the top sheet. Cover the person with a towel or light blanket. Keep all of the body covered during the bed bath, uncovering only one area at a time while washing it.

9. Now have the person lie almost flat.

10. Use one washcloth for soap, one for rinsing, and a dry towel. Have the washcloth very damp, but not dripping.

11. Very gently wash the face first; pat dry, then work your way down the body.

165

NOTE Always start washing at the cleanest part and work toward the dirtiest part.

The Basin Bath

If the person in your care can be in a chair or wheelchair, you can give a sponge bath at the sink. Refer to bed bath, above, for steps on cleansing the person in your care.

The Tub Bath

If the person in your care has good mobility and is strong enough to get in and out of the tub, he or she may enjoy a tub bath. Be sure there are grab bars, a bath bench, and a rubber mat so the person doesn't slide. (It may be easier to sit at bench level rather than at the bottom of the tub.). Refer to bed bath, above, for steps on cleansing the person in your care.

Tip

BATHING IN THE TUB
If a bath bench is not used, many people feel more secure if they turn on to their side and then get on their knees before rising from the tub. This is a very helpful way to get out of the tub if the person is unsteady. Also, remind her to use the grab bars while getting out the tub.

The Shower

Before starting, be sure the shower floor is not slippery. Also make sure there are grab bars, a bath bench, and a rubber mat so the person doesn't slide. A removable shower head is also useful.

Nail Care

When providing nail care, you can watch for signs of irritation or infection. This is especially important in a person with diabetes, for whom a small infection can develop into something more serious. Fingernails and toenails can thicken with age, which will make them more difficult to trim.

1. Assemble supplies—soap, basin with water, towel, nailbrush, scissors, nail clippers, file, and lotion.

2. Wash your hands.

3. Wash the hands of the person in your care with soap and water and soak the hands in a basin of warm water for 5 minutes.

4. Gently scrub the nails with the brush to remove trapped dirt.

5. Dry the nails and gently push back the skin around the nails (the cuticle) with the towel.

6. To prevent ingrown nails, cut nails straight across.

7. File gently to smooth the edges.

8. Gently massage the person's hands and feet with lotion.

 If other members of the household are using the same equipment, clean the nail clippers with alcohol.

Shaving

Shaving can be done by the person in your care, or you can shave his whiskers with a safety razor or an electric razor, however, you should never use an electric razor if the person is on oxygen. If he wears dentures, make sure they are in his mouth.

If the person in your care is on a blood thinner, such as aspirin or Coumadin, be very careful not to knick him. If this happens, you may need to apply pressure with a piece of toilet tissue until the bleeding stops. If bleeding continues, seek medical attention.

Oral Care

Oral care includes cleaning the mouth and gums and the teeth or dentures. Always be patient and explain what you are about to do. (The person who refuses to brush his teeth can swish and spit out a fluoridated mouthwash rinse.)

Oral Care for Someone Who Is Terminally Ill

If your doctor or nurse approves, use hydrogen peroxide diluted with mouthwash or a glycerin/water solution for mouth rinsing. Plain water is best for those who are very sensitive. Your pharmacist can give advice on a gentle mouthwash.

1. Gather supplies—disposable gloves, Toothettes® (foam mouth-swabs), mouthwash, warm water in a glass, and a bowl.

2. Cleanse the mouth (roof, tongue, lips, and cheeks) with the disposable toothbrush.

3. Swab the mouth with a Toothette® dipped in water and repeat until the foam is gone.

4. If the lips are dry, apply a light coat of Vaseline.

Denture Cleaning

1. Remove the dentures from the mouth.

2. Run them under water and soak them in cleaner in a denture cup.

3. Rinse the person's mouth with water or mouthwash.

4. Stimulate (massage) the gums with a very soft toothbrush.

5. Return the dentures to the person's mouth.

 Even a person with dentures should have the soft tissues of the mouth checked regularly by a dentist.

Foot Care

For the comfort and good health of the person in your care:

- Provide properly fitting low-heeled shoes that close with Velcro® or elastic and have nonslip soles. Avoid shoes with heavy soles, running shoes with rubber tips over the toes, and shoes with thick cushioning.

- Provide cotton socks rather than acrylic.

- Trim the person's nails only after a bath when they have softened.

- Use a disposable sponge-tipped toothbrush to clean or dry between the toes.

- Check feet daily for bumps, cuts, and red spots.

Call the doctor or other health care provider if a sore develops on the foot. The person who is diabetic must have special foot care to prevent infections. Serious infections may result in the amputation of a foot.

Foot pain can cause a person to lean back on the heels and increases the chance of a fall, so keep toenails trimmed and feet healthy.

Common Leg and Foot Problems and Solutions

Problem	Solution
Foot strain	Visit a podiatrist.
Calluses	Rub lanolin or lotion on the area; do not cut hard skin.
Cramps	Relieve by movement and massage.
Hammer toes and bunions	Wedge a pad between the big toe and the second toe to straighten them; cut holes in the shoe to relieve rubbing.
Leg ulcers (openings in the skin)	Follow the doctor's instructions. Exercise to keep the foot and ankle mobile.
Swollen legs	Follow the doctor's instructions for treatment of the underlying cause.
Varicose veins	Elevate the legs twice a day for 30 minutes. Before lowering the legs, apply an elastic bandage or stocking.

 Sometimes heart failure patients have chronically swollen legs. Ask your health care provider to prescribe support stockings to alleviate some of this swelling.

Dressing

Dressing a person with disabilities can be made easier by following a routine. Before you begin, lay the clothes out in the order in which they will be put on.

- Dress the person while he or she is sitting.

- Use adaptive equipment like a dressing stick and shoehorn.

- Use loose clothes that are easy to put on and have elastic waistbands, Velcro® fasteners, and front openings.

- Use bras that open and close in front.

- Use tube socks.

- For a person who is confined to bed, use a gown that closes in the back. This will make it easier when using a bedpan or urinal.

 For a person who is confined to bed, be sure to smooth out all wrinkles in the clothes and bedding to prevent pressure sores.

Toileting

Always wear disposable gloves when helping with toileting. This prevents the spread of disease. Wash your hands before and after providing care.

Using a Urinal

1. If the person can't do so himself, place the penis into the urinal as far as possible and hold it in.

2. When the person signals he is finished, remove and empty the urinal.

3. Wash his hands.

4. Wash your own hands.

Using a Commode

A portable commode is helpful for a person with limited mobility. The portable commode (with the pail removed) can be used over the toilet seat and as a shower seat.

Using a Portable Commode

1. Gather the portable commode, toilet tissue, a basin, a cup of water, a washcloth or paper towel, soap, and a towel.

2. Wash your hands.

3. Help the person onto the commode.

4. Offer toilet tissue when the person is finished.

5. Pour a cup of warm water on female genitalia.

6. Pat the area dry with a paper towel.

7. Offer a washcloth so the person can wash his or her hands.

8. Remove the pail from under the seat, empty it, rinse it with clear water, and empty the water into the toilet.

9. Wash your hands.

TOILET SAFETY

Use Velcro® with tape on the back and attach it to the back of the toilet or commode seat to keep the lid from falling.

Using the Bathroom Toilet

If the mobile person is missing the toilet, get a toilet seat in a color that is different from the floor color. This may help him see the toilet better. If he is failing to cleanse the anal area or failing to wash his hands, use tact to encourage him to do so. This will help prevent the spread of infections.

Incontinence

Incontinence is the leakage of urine or a bowel movement over which the person has no control. In addition to bladder management medications, treatments can include bladder training, exercises to strengthen the pelvic floor (Kegel exercises), biofeedback, surgery, electrical muscle stimulator, urinary catheter, prosthetic devices, or external collection devices. Talk to the doctor about the options or treatments for the person in your care.

 Heart failure patients are on medications called diuretics (also known as "water pills"), which may cause them to have to urinate on a urgent basis or more often. This is something to be mindful of because it can potentially lead to an accident, and not be due to incontinence.

To Manage Incontinence:

- Avoid alcohol, coffee, spicy foods, and citrus foods. These can irritate the bladder and can increase the need to urinate.

- Give fluids at regular intervals to dilute the urine. This decreases the irritation of the bladder.

- Be sure the person in your care voids (goes to the bathroom) regularly, ideally every 2 to 3 hours. Use an alarm clock to keep track of the time.

- Provide clothing that can be easily removed.

- Keep a bedpan or a portable commode near the person.

- Provide absorbent products (adult diapers) to be worn under clothes.

- Stroke or tap the lower abdomen to cause voiding.

- Keep the skin dry and clean. Urine on the skin can cause pressure sores and infection.

- Your patience and understanding will help the person have confidence and self-respect.

 NOTE A precise diagnosis for incontinence must be made in order to come up with an effective treatment plan. If the primary care doctor cannot solve the problem, consult an experienced urologist.

Urinary Tract Infection

Urinary tract infection may be present if the person has any of the following signs or symptoms:

- blood in the urine

- a burning feeling when voiding

- cloudy urine with sediment (matter that settles to the bottom)

- pain in the lower abdomen or lower back

- fever and chills

- foul-smelling urine

- a frequent, strong urge to void or frequent voiding

Get in touch with the doctor if there is any sign of a urinary tract infection.

Optimal Bowel Function

Maintaining good bowel function can be a challenge, especially in individuals who are unable to get out of bed and get little exercise. For optimal bowel function—

- Set a time for bowel movements every day or every other day. The best time is 20–30 minutes after breakfast.

- Serve fruits, vegetables, and bran.

- Be sure the person in your care drinks 2 quarts (8 glasses) of water daily (or an amount directed by the doctor). Though water is essential for bowel function, most heart failure patients are on fluid restriction. Make sure to check with the doctor on the amount the person in your care should be drinking.

- Provide a chance for daily exercise.

- Use a stool softener or bulk agent if the stools are too hard. When using a bulk laxative, be sure that 6 to 8 glasses of water are taken per day. This will lessen the chance of severe constipation.

- Use glycerin suppositories as needed to help lubricate the bowels for ease of movement.

- Massage the abdomen in a clockwise direction. This can stimulate a bowel movement.

- Avoid laxatives and enemas unless specifically ordered by the doctor or nurse.

Hemorrhoids

Hemorrhoids are swollen inflamed veins around the anus. They cause tenderness, pain, and bleeding. To treat hemorrhoids, you should do the following:

175

- Be sure to keep anal area clean with premoistened tissues.

- Apply zinc oxide or petroleum jelly to the area.

- Relieve itching by using cold compresses on the anus for 10 minutes several times a day.

- Ask the doctor about suppositories.

Call the Doctor

- if blood from the hemorrhoids is dark red or brown and heavy

- if bleeding continues for more than one week

- if bleeding seems to occur for no reason

Control of Infection in the Home

Common health practices such as frequent hand-washing are necessary to avoid the risk of bacterial, viral, and fungal infections.

> **NOTE** To minimize the chance of infection
> - Always start with the cleanest area and work toward the dirtiest area.
> - Always wash your hands before and after contact with the person in your care and with other people.
> - Always wear disposable gloves when giving personal care.
> - Always wash hands well when returning from a trip outside the house.
> - Always wash your hands after using the toilet.

Cleaning Techniques

The following techniques will help cut the chance of infection in the home.

Caregiver Hand-washing

- Hand-washing is the single most effective way to prevent the spread of infection or germs.

- Use bottle-dispensed hand soap.

- If the person in your care has an infection, use antimicrobial soap.

- Rub your hands for at least 30 seconds to produce lots of lather. Do this away from running water so that the lather is not washed away.

- Use a nailbrush on your nails; keep nails trimmed.

- Wash front and back of hands, between fingers, and at least 2 inches up your wrists.

- Repeat the process.

- Dry your hands on a clean towel or a paper towel.

Skin Care and Prevention of Pressure Sores

Pressure sores (also called decubiti, or bedsores) are blisters or breaks in the skin. They are caused when the body's weight presses blood out of a certain area. The best treatment of pressure sores is prevention. How much time they take to heal depends on how advanced they are.

Facts

- The most common areas for sores are the bony areas— tailbone, hips, heels, and elbows.

- Sores can appear when the skin keeps rubbing on a sheet.

- The skin breakdown starts from the inside, works up to the surface, and can happen in just 15 minutes.

- Damage can range from a change in color in unbroken skin to deep wounds down to the muscle or bone.

- For people with light skin in the first stage of a bedsore, the skin color may change to dark purple or red that does not turn pale under fingertip pressure. For people with dark skin, this area may become darker than normal.

- The affected area may feel warmer than the skin around it.

- Pressure sores that are not treated can lead to hospitalization and can require skin grafts.

Prevention

- Check the skin daily. (Bath time is the ideal time to do this.)

- Provide a well-balanced diet, with enough vitamin C, zinc, and protein.

- Keep the skin dry and clean (urine left on the skin can cause sores and infection).

- Keep clothing loose.

- If splints or braces are used, make sure they are adjusted properly.

- Massage the body with light pressure, using equal parts surgical spirit and glycerin. (Ask a nurse or a pharmacist for advice.)

- Turn a person who is unable to get out of bed at least every 2 hours. Change the person's positions. Smooth wrinkles out of sheets.

- Lightly tape foam to bony sections of the body using paper tape, which will not hurt the skin when peeled off.

- Use flannel or 100% cotton sheets to absorb moisture.

- Provide an egg-crate or sheepskin mattress pad for added comfort.

- Avoid using a plastic sheet or a Chux if they cause sweating.

- When the person is sitting, encourage changing the body position every 15 minutes.

- Use foam pads on chair seats to cushion the buttocks.

- Change the type of chair the person sits in; try an open-back garden chair occasionally.

- Provide as much exercise as possible.

WOUND PREVENTION

If a person tends to scratch or pick at a spot, have the person wear cotton gloves. (Make sure the hands are clean and dry before putting the gloves on.)

Treatment

If you see pressure sores in your daily checking of the skin, you must alert the nurse or the doctor. General guidelines for treatment of these sores are as follows:

- To reduce the chance of infection, wear disposable gloves at all times when providing care.

- Take pressure off sores by changing the person's position often. Use pillows or a foam pad with at least 1 inch of padding to support the body.

- Do not position the person on his or her bony parts.

- Do not let the person lie on pressure sores.

- In bed, change the person's position at least every 2 hours.

- Follow the doctor's or nurse's treatment plan in applying medication to sores and bandaging the areas to protect them while they heal.

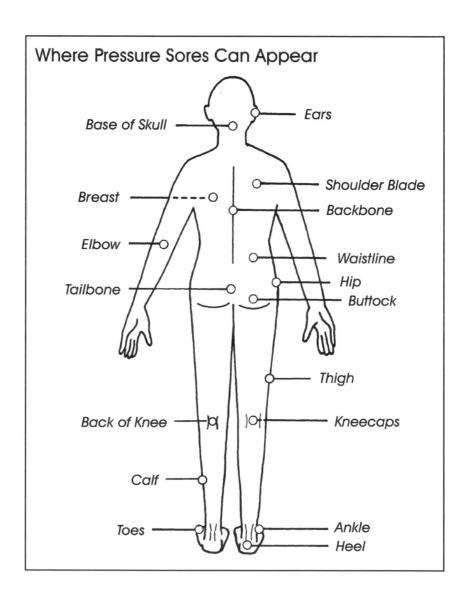

Where Pressure Sores Can Appear

Base of Skull

Ears

Breast

Shoulder Blade

Backbone

Elbow

Waistline

Hip

Tailbone

Buttock

Thigh

Back of Knee

Kneecaps

Calf

Toes

Ankle

Heel

Eating

Mealtimes are important because they provide a welcome break in the day. If it is not too distracting for the person in your care, meals can be eaten with the family. It is important that mealtimes be enjoyable so that the person will look forward to eating.

Look for these free or low-cost solutions:

Community meals—local meal programs sponsored by the federal government and open to those over 59 and their spouses. Call the local Area Agency on Aging or Department of Health and Human Resources.

Meals-on-Wheels—hot meals delivered to the home. Call the Visiting Nurse Association.

Food stamps—help based on income that can stretch food dollars. Call the Department of Health and Human Resources or the Area Agency on Aging.

For best results at mealtime:

- Allow 30 to 45 minutes for eating.

- Avoid fussy meal presentation.

- Make sure all items are ready to eat and within reach.

- Provide a comfortable table and chair or other eating arrangement.

- Supply easy-to-hold eating utensils. To avoid cuts, throw out all chipped cups and plates.

- Reduce excess noise such as TV and radio.

- If the person's vision is poor, place the same foods in the same spot on the plate every time.

Boosting Food Intake When the Appetite Is Poor

- Offer more food at the time of day when the person is most hungry or less tired.

- To increase the appeal of food for those with decreased taste and smell, provide strong flavors.

- Use milk or cream instead of water in soups and cooked cereal.

- Add nonfat dry-milk powder to foods like yogurt, mashed potatoes, gravy, and sauces.

- Offer milk or fruit shakes.

(📖 See **Diet, Nutrition, and Exercise,** Chapter 15)

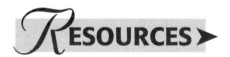

Meeting Life's Challenges
9042 Aspen Grove Lane
Madison, WI 53717
Fax (608) 824-0403
www.meetinglifeschallenges.com
E-mail: help@meetinglifeschallenges.com
Offers a guide called Dressing Tips and Clothing Resources for Making Life Easier, by Shelley P. Schwarz, a guide to dressing for people with disabilities plus more than 100 resources for custom clothing.

National Association for Continence (NAFC)
P.O. Box 8310
Spartanburg, SC 29305-8310
(800) 252-3337; (864) 579-7900; Fax (864) 579-7902
www.nafc.org
NAFC is a leading source of education and support to the public about the diagnosis, treatments, and management alternatives for incontinence.

If you don't have home access to the Internet, ask your local library to help you locate any Web site.

Therapies

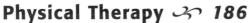

Therapies

*T*he following information is provided for your general knowledge. It is NOT a substitute for training with professional therapists. Medicare, Medicaid and private insurances may cover physical and occupational therapy either in the home or in an outpatient setting. Cardiac rehabilitation may be covered as well. You can check with your insurance about benefits for these services. If the person in your care is hospitalized, the discharge planner can determine if there is coverage and arrange this.

Physical Therapy

Physical therapy is part of the process of relearning how to function after an injury, illness, or period of inactivity. If muscles are not used, they shorten and tighten, making joint motion painful.

What a Physical Therapist Does

A physical therapist treats a person to relieve pain, build up and restore muscle function, and maintain the best possible performance. The therapist does this by using physical means such as active and passive exercise, massage, heat, water, and electricity. Broadly speaking, a physical therapist:

• sets up the goals of treatment with patient and family

• shows how to use special equipment

• instructs in routine daily functions

- teaches safe ways to move

- sets up and teaches an exercise program

 The American Physical Therapy Association, often located in the state capital, can provide a list of licensed therapists.

What a Physical Therapist Determines

Depending on a person's physical condition, a therapist may work on range-of-motion exercises, correct body positions when resting, devices to help the person in your care, and other simple ways to improve daily functions.

A physical therapist checks things that can affect a person's daily activities—

- the person's attitude toward his situation

- how well he can move his muscles and joints (range of motion)

- his ability to see, smell, hear, and feel

- what he can do on his own and what he needs to learn

- his equipment needs, now and in the future

- what can be improved in the home to make moving around safer and more comfortable

- who can and will help to give support

Range-of-Motion (ROM) Exercises

The purpose of range-of-motion exercises is to relieve pain, maintain normal body alignment (positions), help prevent skin swelling and breakdown, and promote bone formation.

Joints Used in ROM

▲ shoulder

▲ hip

▲ feet, ankle, toe

▲ hands

▲ wrists

▲ elbows

▲ shoulders

▲ finger/thumb

▲ neck

A ROM exercise program should be started before deformities develop. Here are some things to do when you are asked to help with exercises at home:

- Communicate what you are doing.

- Use the flats of both hands, not the fingertips, to hold a body part.

- Take each movement only as far as the joint will go into a comfortable stretch. (Mild discomfort is okay, but it should go away quickly.)

- Do each exercise 3 to 5 times.

- Use slow steady movements to help relax muscles and increase joint range.

- If joints are swollen and painful, exercise very gently.

Occupational Therapy

Occupational therapy is designed to help people regain and build skills that are important for functioning on their own. The occupational therapist will help the person evaluate levels of function.

The occupational therapist will—

- test a person's strength, range of motion, endurance (the ability to continue an activity or effort), and dexterity (skill in using hands) to do everyday tasks that were done easily before an illness or injury happened

- design a program of activities and solutions that ensure the greatest possible independence

- provide training to relearn everyday activities of daily living like eating, grooming, dressing, toileting, bathing, and leisure activities

- decide whether special equipment is needed, such as wheelchairs, feeding devices, transfer equipment, hand and skin devices

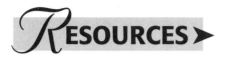

RESOURCES ➤

American Heart Association
7272 Greenville Avenue
Dallas, TX 75231
Phone: (214) 373-6300 or
1-800-AHA-USA1
www.amhrt.org

The American Association of Cardiovascular and Pulmonary Rehabilitation (AACVPR)
http://www.aacvpr.org/certification/program_cert_search.cfm
Offers a list of available cardiac rehabilitation programs in all states.

American Horticultural Therapy Association
3570 E. 12th Avenue, Suite 206
Denver, CO 80206
(800) 634-1603; Fax (303) 322-2485
www.ahta.org
Support and education resource for people interested in horticultural therapy.

Delta Society
875 124th Avenue NE, Suite 101
Bellevue, WA 98005
(425) 226-7357; Fax (425) 235-1076
www.deltasociety.org
E-Mail: info@deltasociety.org
Provides information on the human-animal bond and information on how to obtain a service animal.

National Center of Complementary and Alternative Medicine Clearinghouse
(888) 644-6226
www.nccam.nih.gov
For more information on garden hints, call your local county office of the **Home Extension Service**.

Contact your local **Humane Society** for information about pet therapy.

If you don't have home access to the Internet, ask your local library to help you locate any Web site.

Special Challenges

Special Challenges

Communication

Communication is the ability to speak, understand speech, read, write, and gesture. Nonverbal messages are given through silence, body movements, or facial expression. Be aware that words can carry one message, the body another.

To communicate better with the person in your care, try:

• helping the person communicate frustrations

• pacing activities, because the person will tire easily

Improving the Chance of Being Understood

When talking to a person with hearing loss, follow these guidelines:

• Sit in the light so your lips and facial expressions can be seen.

• Make eye contact.

• Use body language (nodding, pointing) and lots of facial expression.

• Speak louder without shouting. Shouting makes words more difficult to understand.

Depression

Changes in mood are common in people with chronic medical conditions, such as congestive heart failure. The person in your care may show signs of sad or depressed mood and anxiety. These symptoms often worsen as her medical condition worsens. You will probably find that on days when she feels physically worse her mood will probably be lower. An occasional change in mood doesn't mean that someone is depressed, but it is important to pay attention when a sad or "blue" mood continues.

Listed below are the signs/symptoms of depression:

- persistent sad, anxious or "empty" mood

- feelings of hopelessness, pessimism

- feelings of guilt, worthlessness, helplessness

- loss of interest or pleasure in hobbies and activities that were once enjoyed, including sex

- decreased energy, fatigue, being "slowed down"

- difficulty concentrating, remembering, making decisions

- insomnia, early-morning awakening, middle of the night awakening or oversleeping

- appetite and/or weight changes

- thoughts of death or suicide, or suicidal attempts

- restlessness, irritability

It is important to seek treatment for depression. Depression doesn't just go away. It will worsen without treatment. The most effective ways of treating depression are counseling and/or medication. Depression is a real, physical symptom, and it responds well to treatment. It's important to think about depression like other medical problems, such as high blood pressure and diabetes. It's not possible to just think depression away. People often don't want to think about receiving treatment for depression, saying things like "I am not crazy." In addition to medication, counseling can also be helpful. Medicare, Medicaid, and private insurance often cover the cost of counseling (there may be a co-pay). Remember, it is important to seek treatment for depression; it won't go away by itself. Talk about symptoms of depression with your doctor.

 Depression is often misdiagnosed as dementia or Alzheimer's, so be aware that medications and progressive heart failure often affect memory. Memory changes can also be a symptom of depression.

Sexual Expression

Sexual interest and performance often diminish in people with heart failure. This can be due to medications and the progression of the disease. The changes don't mean a loss of sexuality. The needs for intimacy and sharing do not change, although the ability to perform or respond in the usual manner may. To improve your spouse's or partner's ability to exercise sexual expression, try to increase self-esteem and downplay the role of "patient." It may be helpful to discuss these concerns with your health care provider.

Common Fears of a Person with a Chronic Illness

- loss of self-image
- loss of control over life
- loss of independence and fear of abandonment
- fear of living alone and being lonely
- fear of death

You can help deal with these powerful emotions by:

- pointing out the person's strengths and focusing on small successes

- restoring areas of control to the person by giving as many choices as possible and having the person manage as much of their self-care as possible

- finding new ways for the person to adjust to limitations

- providing insight into sources of meaning in life

- changing your attitude about the person's disability

- recognizing that humor is healing and providing large doses of laughter to stimulate a positive attitude, providing humorous books, comics, cartoons, television, or movies

- allowing the person to cry, realizing that it is a way of coping with illness

- allowing for the power of silence

- providing opportunities for peer support and friendship (which works exceptionally well with the elderly)

Seasonal Affective Disorder

Some depression can be brought on by the dark, gloomy days of winter. This type of depression may be treated by sitting in front of full-spectrum lights for one hour per day. However, be wary of gadgets that promise miraculous results.

Dealing with Boredom

Boredom is another problem for people who are ill, and fighting it can take all your creativity. Try—

- watching funny movies

- taking car rides; try to get out of the house each day

- listening to music, especially from the person's youth

- taking up hobbies

- interacting with friends and family

- playing board games and card games

- attending public library discussion clubs

- spending time with others in similar difficulties—in religious groups, recreation centers, or the YMCA/ YWCA

- being involved in volunteer service organizations such as the Mended Hearts (see **Resource** section)

- using a computer and accessing sites on the Internet (which helps prevent loneliness through interesting activity and provides the ability to communicate with family and friends through e-mail)

- attending continuing education classes at local colleges or correspondence schools can provide education opportunities, even for shut-ins. There are opportunities for both academic and nonacademic classes (for example, boat building, ceramics, and garden design).

TUITION DISCOUNTS

Some states are encouraging older students to attend college by offering tuition discounts at public institutions.

The Internet and Computers

Consider a computer for the person in your care. A computer is ideal for the person who has difficulty writing.

Computer software is available that helps users who are visually impaired, deaf, or have other disabilities.

TECHNOLOGY
Check the local library for computers classes or for help locating any Web sites.

Working with Heart Failure

A person newly diagnosed with heart failure, whose symptoms are well controlled, may be able to continue to work. The type of work a person performs will also affect the ability to maintain employment. If someone has a job where they are sitting much of the day, she might be able to continue working longer than someone who has a job with more physical demands. For example, someone who works at a dry cleaner, standing all day in a warm setting, may find it very hard to continue to work. However, the heart failure patient who works at a desk in a comfortable temperature may be able to continue job responsibilities for some time. Transportation to and from work may also influence the ability to continue work. Someone who rides a bus and then has to walk several blocks may find it difficult because of swollen legs or shortness of breath. Some employers may be willing to adjust daily responsibilities to accommodate the person's needs, for example, the person who works on a factory assembly line may be able to change his work task and be in an office setting.

However, as heart failure progresses, most people have to stop working. This may come at a time when some people would be ready to retire, so the change happens when she no longer expected to work. She might be at the age when she will qualify for Social Security and Medicare benefits. For others, this decision is made earlier than they expected. This can be very difficult decision because work is an important part of life, and there can be a sense of loss at giving up a job. It is yet another example of how illness has impacted her life. Financial concerns also play a part in the decision to stop working. It is important for you and the person in your care to talk with each other and with your primary care doctor or cardiologist about this important decision. Sometimes physicians are more effective at discussing work responsibilities. They may be concerned about the patient's worsening heart failure and how continuing to work may affect the patient's condition in a negative way. If your physician doesn't start the conversation about work, then ask her opinion.

If he has paid into the Social Security system, he may be eligible for Social Security Disability (SSD) or Supplemental Security Income (SSI). To begin this process, contact his local Social Security office. There will be paperwork for him to complete, and he will need to provide medical records from his doctors. Many employees are covered under their employer's disability insurance, and veterans should contact their local Veterans Administration to determine if they may be eligible for benefits.

Pain Management

Pain is an individual experience that is tied to both physical and mental states. Even noise makes a person tense, which can contribute to pain. Fatigue, depression, and anxiety can make pain harder to tolerate. (Lying in bed does not lessen the pain, although it may appear that the person is comfortable and relaxed.)

Types of Pain

Pain falls into two categories:

Acute—short-term pain from illness or injury, which can be managed with prescribed narcotics and will subside when the injury heals

Chronic—pain that begins with an illness, is long term (more than six months), and is controlled with medications, which may create other problems as the tolerance of those medications increases

Pain Reduction Techniques

The most effective methods for relieving pain are pain medications (analgesics), sleep, immobilization, and distraction. (Also, heat and cold increase or decrease circulation to the affected area, but should not be used without specific instructions from a doctor.)

To reduce pain, consider:

- distraction through TV, music, or reading aloud

- distraction from a medical procedure by massaging the person's hand

- reduction of stress and promotion of healing through relaxation, meditation, and prayer

 NOTE Although good nutrition will not relieve pain, it promotes healing by strengthening the body.

Pain can be controlled through the following techniques:

- **Biofeedback**—the monitoring of reactions to conscious and subconscious thoughts by measuring changes in blood pressure, temperature, and body organs

- **Deep Breathing**—slow deep breaths taken through the nose and exhaled slowly through pursed lips (relieves pain by increasing oxygen to brain)

- **Hypnosis**—an altered state of consciousness that replaces a focus on pain with attention to another idea

- **Meditation**—a technique for visualizing relief from pain

- **Surgery**—permanent severing of nerves to block pain (a step that requires careful consideration)

- **Topical Pain Relievers**—creams, rubs, or sprays applied to muscles or joints for pain relief in a specific area

 NOTE Sound sleep is often interrupted for people with heart failure. They may become short of breath at night or may have to urinate frequently. When a person does not sleep well at night, expect more naps during the day.

Abuse

Abusive behavior is never acceptable. Though tensions can mount in the most loving families and result in frustration and anger, an emotionally damaging or physically forceful response is not okay. When this happens, call for a time-out, and call for help. If a home health agency is involved, you may also contact them. The physician for the person in your care is another person to call for help. If concerned about your own safety, or that of the person in your care, you may need to call an emergency number in your community, like the local police department.

Physical abuse usually begins in the process of giving or receiving personal help. For instance, the caregiver might be too rough during dressing or grooming, or the person receiving care might accidentally scratch the caregiver during a transfer. Once anger and frustration reach this level, abuse by either person may become frequent.

The dangers of physical abuse are easy to see, but emotional abuse is also unhealthy and damaging. Continued shaming, harsh criticism, or controlling behaviors can damage the self-esteem of either person.

Dealing with Anger and Elder Abuse

Communicating When the Person in Your Care Is Angry

To help diffuse a situation so that it doesn't become a problem, here is how to communicate with someone who is angry.

DO

- Be patient, calm, courteous, sympathetic, and show your concern and caring.

- Be open to listening to the person explain the problem before you respond with an answer.

- Look at the problem from the point of view of the person in your care.

- Remember, the person is upset about a situation, not you.

DON'T

- Be defensive and angry.

- Raise your voice (yelling never helps).

- Intimidate the person in your care. It is important that you, as caregiver, manage your anger. Ask, "What can we do to make things better?" Think about your own feelings and what button is being pushed. Understanding what is upsetting you will help you from losing control.

Tips You Can Use to Diffuse Anger

1. Communicate. Tell the person in your care that you understand or are trying to. "If it happened to me, I'd be angry too."

2. Remind the person that she has choices. Because of her anger she may not realize the choices she has.

3. Affirm her feelings. Say, "I see you are angry."

4. Repeat yourself like a broken record. Softly repeat what is necessary.

What You Can Do

Help the person in your care identify a trusted person who can be called on for help. The Adult Protective Services Agency—a component of the human service agency in most states—is typically responsible for investigating reports of domestic abuse and providing families with help and guidance. Other professionals who may be able to help include doctors or nurses, police officers, lawyers, and social workers.

If you suspect abuse in an institutional setting, such as a nursing home, report concerns to your state long-term-care ombudsman.

Each state has such an ombudsman program to investigate and address nursing-home complaints. The National Center on Elder Abuse Web site maintains a list of phone numbers, by state, which you can call for assistance if you suspect domestic or institutional elder abuse. Visit www.elderabusecenter.org. If someone you care about is in imminent danger, call 911, police, or hospital emergency NOW.

Signs of Abuse

Knowing the signs and symptoms of abuse can help you determine if there is a problem.

Signs and symptoms may include:

- Physical injury—bruises, cuts, burns or rope marks, broken bones or sprains that can't be explained.

- Emotional abuse—feeling of helplessness, a hesitation to talk openly, fear, withdrawal, depression, feelings of denial or agitation.

- Lack of physical care—malnourishment, weight loss, poor hygiene, as well as bedsores, soiled bedding, unmet medical needs.

- Unusual behaviors—changes in the person's behavior or emotional state such as withdrawal, fear, or anxiety, apathy.

- Changes in living arrangements.

- Unexplained changes such as the appearance of previously uninvolved relatives or newly met strangers moving in.

- Financial changes—missing money or valuables, unexplained financial transactions, unpaid bills despite available funds, and sudden transfer of assets.

Be alert to the senior's comments about being taken advantage of.

NOTE As many as 1.2 million seniors have been abused at some point in their lives. Those most at risk of being abused are people who suffer from dementia.
Source: American Geriatrics Society.

Transportation and Travel

Transportation

There is a network of transportation services, public and private, that will pick up the disabled and the elderly at their homes. These services rely on vans and paid drivers and run on a schedule to specific locations. Free transportation is available from community volunteer organizations, although most public services charge on a sliding scale.

 NOTE Many states ensure transportation to necessary medical care for Medicaid/Medicare recipients. Check with your local Medicaid/Medicare office to see if you qualify.

Community transportation services are provided by:

- home health care agencies
- public health departments
- religious organizations
- civic clubs
- the local American Red Cross
- the Area Agency on Aging
- local public transportation companies

Traveling with Medications

Traveling with medications should not stop you and your care receiver from enjoying travel. Here are some tips when traveling with medications:

- Bring enough medication to last through your trip plus some extras.

- Pack your meds in a carry-on bag—luggage can stray or become lost.

- Keep all medication in original containers with original prescription labels.

- Make a list of the medications the person takes, and why, with brand and generic names. Make a copy and pack one copy separately.

- Make arrangements for refrigerating the medication.

- If intravenous medication is used, carry a used-needle container.

- Bring the person insurance ID card, plus instructions for accessing a physician where you are going.

- Bring the doctor name and contact information, in case of emergency.

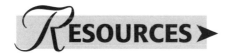

RESOURCES ➤

Abuse

National Center for Elder Abuse (NCEA)
1201 15th Street, NW
Suite 350
Washington, DC 20005-2842
(202) 898-2586
Fax (202) 898-2583
www.elderabusecenter.org
Offers fact sheets, reporting numbers, news, publications, and resources.

Mended Hearts
1-800-AHA-USA1 or 1-800-242-8721
www.mendedhearts.org
This is a nationwide patient support organization for people with heart disease, their families, medical professionals and other interested people.

Pain Management Resources

The National Chronic Pain Outreach Association
P.O. Box 274
Millboro, VA 24460
(540) 862-9437 Fax: (540)862-9485
www.chronicpain.org
E-mail: ncpoa@cfw.com
A membership organization that offers a quarterly newsletter (Lifeline), a catalogue of related publications, national physician referrals, and support group listings. Membership is $25 per year.

The Worldwide Congress on Pain
http://www.pain.com

If you don't have home access to the Internet, ask your local library to help you locate any Web site.

Diet, Nutrition, and Exercise

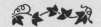

Diet, Nutrition, and Exercise

*F*ollowing dietary guidelines and recommendations is very important for the person with heart failure. Controlling sodium and fluid intake can reduce chances of being hospitalized and help improve functioning in the home. Heart failure is not going to go away, but it is important for both you, the caregiver, and the person in your care to control what can be controlled. What the person in your care eats is her responsibility, but the caregiver can help by purchasing and preparing low-salt, heart healthy foods.

Older heart failure patients need fewer calories to maintain normal body weight. Their bodies absorb fewer nutrients so they must eat high-nutrient food to maintain good health. They must get more nutrients from less food. If a person does not get enough calories, the body will use stored nutrients for energy. When this happens, the person becomes weaker and is more likely to get infections.

Check with the doctor before starting any special diets. Also, check with a doctor, pharmacist, or registered dietitian to know what effect prescription medicines have on nutritional needs.

NOTE Use every means possible to perk up the appetite, especially since most heart failure patients feel their food "has no taste" without salt. Make sure the person's dentures fit correctly and that his glasses are adequate. We eat with our eyes before we ever touch our food.

Careful Food Preparation

Food preparation and eating are often considered social activities, so it is helpful for all members of the family to understand the diet recommendations for the person in your care. Dietary changes are much easier when the whole family follows them.

Individuals with a chronic medical problem are especially susceptible to illness from unsafe food, so be extra careful when preparing their meals.

- Wash your own hands and the hands of the person in your care with antibacterial soap before preparing or serving food.

- Dry hands with a paper towel.

- Disinfect the sink and kitchen counters with a solution of 1 teaspoon chlorine bleach per liter of water. (Save the solution for just one week because it loses strength.)

- Air drying dishes is more sanitary than using a dish towel.

- Check expiration dates carefully, and discard all meats that are past the expiration date on the label.

- Cook all red meat and fish thoroughly.

- Cook hamburgers or chopped meat to an internal temperature of 160° F. (There is much less chance of being infected by a solid piece of meat like a steak or roast because bacteria collects only on the outside of those cuts.)

- Cook meat to at least at an oven temperature of 300° F.

- Keep hot foods hot at 140° F or more and cold foods at 40° F or colder.

- Keep the refrigerator below 41° F.

- Cook eggs until the yolks are no longer runny.

- Don't serve raw eggs in milk shakes or other drinks.

- Don't serve oysters, clams, or shellfish raw.

- Wash all fruits and vegetables thoroughly.

- Avoid unpasteurized milk and cider.

- Do not add salt when preparing food. Some salt substitutes may be used, but check with the doctor or dietitian first, because some may NOT be acceptable.

- Find out what amount of sodium is allowed in the diet of the person in your care.

- Involve the person in your care in meal planning and adapting to a low-sodium diet.

- Learn how to read labels, so you can calculate sodium content when preparing meals.

- Look for low-sodium recipes.

- Serve low-sodium snacks when planning parties, family events, or holiday gatherings.

NOTE If the water temperature is set too low, the dishwasher will not sterilize the dishes.

Nutrition Guidelines for People with Heart Failure

Be aware of salt/sodium guidelines for those with heart failure. Typically, 2 grams or 2,000 milligrams of sodium a day is recommended.

- Make tasty, nutritionally well-balanced meals that promote good bowel function and a normal flow of urine.

- Offer drinking water or liquids at mealtime to make chewing and swallowing easier. However, a person with heart failure will typically be told to limit fluid intake to 2,000 milliliters a day. Two thousand milliliters equals a 2-liter bottle of soda. Any item that is liquid at room temperature should be counted towards fluid intake.

- Avoid lard, bacon fat, coconut and palm kernel oil, sweets, and highly seasoned foods.

- Serve fresh fruits and vegetables. They are good sources of fiber and vitamins A and C, and they prevent constipation.

- Do not serve too much processed food, which lacks fiber and contributes to constipation and sodium intake.

- To improve sluggish appetites, use seasonings like herbs, spices, lemon juice, peppers, garlic, and vinegar, especially since salt is restricted.

Boosting Calorie or Protein Intake

- Offer most of the food when the person is most hungry.

- Add non-fat powdered milk to any food with liquid in it, such as desserts, soups, gravy, and cereal.

- Add cottage cheese or ricotta cheese to casseroles, scrambled eggs, and desserts.

- Grate cheeses on bread, meats, vegetables, eggs, and casseroles. Check the sodium level of cheese, it can be quite high. Look for low-sodium cheeses.

- Use instant breakfast powder in milk drinks and desserts.

- Add nuts (salt-free), seeds, and wheat germ to breads, cereal, casseroles, and desserts.

- Add beaten eggs to mashed potatoes, sauces, vegetable purees, and cooked puddings.

- Add honey, jam, or sugar to bread, milk drinks, fruit, and yogurt desserts.

- Add mayonnaise to salads and sandwiches.

Quick and Easy Snacks

Be sure to first check with your doctor about sugar, salt, or potassium restrictions.

- low-sodium cheese on crackers

- chocolate milk

- fruits, especially ripe bananas

- granola cookies

- hard-boiled eggs

- milkshakes

- puddings

- raisins, nuts, prunes

Dining Out

Pay attention to food selection when eating out at restaurants. Remember that 70 percent of the sodium we eat each day is in food that might not taste salty. Here are few tips to follow when dining out with a person with heart failure:

- When choosing restaurants, avoid places that serve only fried or pre-prepared foods, such as fast food restaurants.

- Ask the waiter to prepare food *without* salt or monosodium glutamate (MSG).

- Bring healthy snacks to places such as movie theaters or sporting events, where foods high in sodium are usually eaten.

- Eat a healthy meal at home before going to an event.

- Save menus from places that deliver low-sodium foods.

- Call ahead to the restaurant or check the Internet for the nutrition information for the menu offered.

Therapeutic Diets

Keep the doctor informed about the diet prepared for the person in your care. A special diet may be prescribed to:

- improve or maintain a person's health

- change the amount of bulk, as in a high-fiber diet

- change the consistency of food, as in a special soft diet

- eliminate or decrease certain foods

- change the number of calories

Osteoporosis Prevention

Many women and even men suffer from osteoporosis, a condition that occurs when minerals are lost from the bones, thereby weakening them to the point where they break easily and are slow to heal.

Osteoporosis can be prevented by:

- getting calcium from dairy foods; leafy vegetables such as kale and collards; broccoli; salmon; and sardines. Check with the doctor about these foods if the person in your care is taking Coumadin, a blood thinner, because these foods can reduce the effects of this medication.

- taking calcium supplements (with vitamin D in the evening because it absorbs during sleep)

- vitamin D also plays an important role in bone health by helping with the calcium absorption. Our bodies can make vitamin D with just 15–20 minutes of skin exposure to the sun each day. Vitamin D can also be found fortified in foods that contain calcium. Be careful with supplementation because vitamin D is stored in the body and can be toxic in relatively low amounts (>2,000 i.u./day).

> **NOTE** The National Institutes of Health recommends that post-menopausal women consume 1,500 milligrams of calcium daily to slow bone loss.

Recommended Daily Allowances for a Person Over Age 51

If you are concerned that the person in your care is malnourished, do a calorie check periodically. Recommended daily allowances are:

- women— 1600–1900 calories per day

- men— 2000–2200 calories per day

Additional Sources of Calcium, Folate, and Protein

The diets of those with chronic illness are often deficient in these nutrients, which are found in the following foods: (*denotes most concentrated sources). Remember to check with your physician regarding sodium and potassium guidelines.

Calcium (one cup serving, except where noted)
Cheddar cheese (1 oz.)
Collards (1/2 cup, cooked)—May need to limit if the person in your care is taking Coumadin.
Lactaid milk, nonfat, calcium fortified*
Milk, skim or 1%
Orange juice, with added calcium*

Ricotta, fat-free (1/4 cup)
Swiss cheese (1 oz.)*
Total® brand cereal (3/4 cup)*
Yogurt, nonfat, plain*

Folate (one cup serving, except where noted)
Brewer's yeast (1 tablespoon)
Chickpeas or pinto beans, cooked
Ensure brand nutrition supplement
Lentils, cooked*
Orange juice
Product 19 brand cereal*
Red kidney beans
Spinach (1/2 cup, cooked)
Total® brand cereal (3/4 cup)*

Protein (4 oz. serving, except where noted)
Beans or peas (1 cup)
Beef steak, eye of round, well trimmed*
Chicken (without skin or bone)*
Chili with beans (1 cup)
Eggs
Flounder*
Lamb, well trimmed*
Lentils (1 cup cooked)*
Pork tenderloin, well trimmed*
Salmon, canned, drained
Tuna, canned in water, drained*
Turkey (without skin or bone)*
Yogurt, nonfat, plain (8 oz.)

NOTE These may not be the best foods for a person under special medical treatment. Special diets and products to improve nutrition should only be used on the advice of a doctor or registered dietitian. Special diets, especially if the person in your care has other medical problems, like diabetes, should be discussed with a doctor or registered dietitian.

Checklist **Nutrition Assessment**

To assess nutrition risk for the person in your care, check the following questions. If the answer to most of the points is Yes, the person is at risk and you need to contact the doctor for a diet. Answer the questions every six months or whenever you notice big changes in weight or eating habits.

✓ Has she recently lost weight? About how much? _____ lbs.

✓ Has she had any recent appetite loss? _____ For how long? _____ (days, weeks, months)

✓ Does she have difficulty chewing? _____

✓ Does she have difficulty swallowing? _____

✓ Food allergies? _____

✓ A special diet? _____

✓ Have you been given instructions about her diet? _____

✓ Does she eat fewer than 2 meals per day? _____

✓ Does she eat few fruits, vegetables, and dairy products? _____

✓ How many servings per day?
Fruits _____
Vegetables _____
Dairy _____

✓ Does she drink more than 3 alcoholic beverages per day? _____

✓ Does she eat most of her meals alone? _____

Weight Loss

This is not a diet book, but if you or the person in your care are overweight, then losing weight will require some change in diet. Whatever diet your doctor recommends, losing weight is a matter of taking in fewer calories than your body burns. It's like balancing a caloric checkbook, where calories are cash and weight is savings.

More calories burned than eaten = decreasing weight
More calories eaten than burned = increasing weight

NOTE If you eat 10 calories more than you burn every day for a year, you'll gain 1 lb—3,600 calories = 1 lb.

If you do that for 20 years—just 10 calories more a day—at the end of 20 years, you'll have gained 20 lbs.

Ten calories is an insignificant amount of food. For many people, they eat more than a hundred extra calories per day. This simple equation may explain why 60 percent of Americans are either overweight or obese.

Diet and Nutrition Education

If you need reliable, well-organized, user-friendly advice about a healthy diet, get a copy of *The No-Fad Diet* from the American Heart Association (AHA). It is the only diet book the AHA has ever written, and it contains all the information you need about diet, exercise, and behavior change. It also contains sample meal plans, easy-to-prepare recipes, and information on starting an exercise program. One of the key features of the book is that it addresses the psychological component of changing behavior. The book is available at the American Heart Association Web site, through online booksellers, or your local bookstore. In addition, AHA offers many cookbooks, all designed to combat cardiovascular disease and stroke.

Cholesterol

Cholesterol is present in the cell wall of every cell in animal bodies, including human animals. The amount of cholesterol determines how permeable (leaky) the cell is. Cholesterol has a couple of other positive roles, but that cell-wall function is the main one. Cholesterol is so important to our basic biology that our bodies manufacture all the cholesterol they need from saturated fat. Dietary cholesterol is extra.

Cholesterol manufacture is under genetic control, and it is possible that diet and exercise won't be enough to lower the numbers of the person in your care. Cholesterol-lowering medication may be called for. Older cholesterol drugs work to block absorption of dietary cholesterol. A new type of drug addresses the manufacture of cholesterol in the liver.

Lowering the intake of *saturated fat* will help lower cholesterol level.

Saturated fat is fat that is solid at room temperature, like butter or the fat on meat.

Unsaturated fat is liquid at room temperature, like vegetable oil. "Good oils" are olive, peanut and corn oil.

To get from your liver to your cells, cholesterol has to travel in your blood. Although technically a kind of fat, cholesterol is like a wax, think egg-yolk residue on a plate after breakfast. Since blood is mostly water, it doesn't know what to do with wax. It can't dissolve it, so it wraps it in protein. That's where cholesterol gets its other name—lipoprotein.

Tip Baffled by the LDL/HDL distinction? Low-density lipoprotein (LDL) is *bad* cholesterol, think L for "lousy." Another easy way to remember this is to think of LDL as "less-desirable lipids." LDL cholesterol doesn't move in liquid as well and tends to be stickier and so sticks to blood vessel walls. High-density lipoprotein (HDL) is the *good* kind, think H for "healthy" or HDL as "highly desirable lipids." HDL tends to flow more freely in the blood stream and is not as sticky.

Whether cholesterol is LDL or HDL is largely determined by activity levels—in other words, you can't eat more or less of either one. To increase HDL levels exercise more.

To reduce dietary cholesterol there has to be decreased intake of animal products. All meat, dairy, and eggs contain some cholesterol, no matter their fat content, because all animal cells contain cholesterol.

In addition, tropical oils (palm and coconut) and partially hydrogenated oils also contribute to cholesterol numbers.

Tip Partially hydrogenated oil is vegetable oil with hydrogen whipped into it, generally to increase shelf life. Nutritionists now label these oils as "trans-fat." It is suspected that trans-fats also contribute to atherosclerosis (a disease in which cholesterol deposits form on the walls of arteries, narrowing them). More restaurants and food products are now trans-fat free, but they still may contain small quantities of partially hydrogenated or hydrogenated oils.

Blood Pressure

Diet affects blood pressure because it affects weight, sodium, and atherosclerosis. Atherosclerosis increases blood pressure by narrowing arteries from the inside. Sodium causes water retention because our kidneys need water to maintain a proper electrolyte balance. This retained water puts pressure on the blood vessels and keeps them from relaxing, thereby increasing blood pressure.

Nutrition scientists have formulated the DASH Diet. (DASH stands for dietary approach to stop hypertension.) The DASH Diet was designed by the National Heart, Lung and Blood Institute after rigorous investigation into which vitamins, minerals, and micronutrients affected blood pressure.

The DASH Diet is low in saturated fat, cholesterol, and total fat. It emphasizes fruits, vegetables, and low-fat dairy foods, and includes whole-grain products, fish, poultry, and nuts. It is reduced in red meat, sweets, and sugar-containing beverages, and is rich in magnesium, potassium, and calcium, as well as protein and fiber. It controls for sodium. Research has reported reductions in blood pressure in as little as two weeks after beginning the DASH diet.

NOTE *Facts about the DASH Eating Plan* is a 24-page booklet that includes a week's worth of recipes. It is published by the National Institutes of Health, NIH Publication 03-4082, May 2003. E-mail nhlbi@prospectassoc.com or call 301592-8573. To view online, go to www.nhlbi.nih.gov and type the booklet's title in the search window.

> Blood pressure is affected by more than one biological/chemical mechanism. In order to control high blood pressure, doctors may prescribe more than one blood pressure medication because different drugs work with different mechanisms. Each pill plays a role in reducing the numbers, as does your diet.

A Foundation of Good Nutrition

Bringing good nutrition to the table takes planning, attention, and some imagination. A foundation to healthy eating can be found in the U.S. Department of Agriculture's *MyPyramid*. Making smart choices from each part of the pyramid is the best way to ensure one's body gets the balanced nutrition it needs. Here are some easy tips to make the most of every food group, and get the most from the calories eaten:

- **Focus on fruits.** Select fresh, frozen, or dried fruits over juices for most of your fruit choices. Avoid canned vegetables because of the high sodium content.

- **Vary your vegetables.** Choose from a rainbow of colors—dark green, such as broccoli, kale, and spinach; orange, such as carrots, pumpkin, and sweet potatoes; yellow, such as yellow peppers and butternut squash. If the person in your care is on a blood thinner, such as Coumadin, she should have a consistent intake of green leafy vegetables. Speak with the doctor or dietitian about this.

- **Try to buy whole-grain products.** When selecting cereals, breads, crackers, or pastas, look to see that the grains listed on the ingredient list are "whole." Whole-grains provide a great source of fiber and can help in managing weight and controlling constipation. "Whole-grain" is not the same as "enriched."

- **Keep it lean.** Choose lean meats, fish, and poultry and bake, broil, or grill whenever possible. Try to vary your protein choices and add or substitute beans, peas, lentils, nuts, and seeds to what you eat.

- **Calcium counts.** Include 3 cups of low-fat or fat-free milk, yogurt, or equivalent of low-fat cheeses every day to maintain good bone health. Calcium-fortified foods and beverages can help fill the gap if you don't or can't consume milk.

- **Limit your fat, sugar, and salt.** These "extras" can add up! Check out the nutrition label on foods and look for foods low in saturated and trans fats. Sugars often only provide added calories with little added nutritional value. Choose and prepare foods with little or no salt or sodium. You can buy low-sodium soups and products that claim there is no salt added, however, it is still important to read labels to check the sodium content.

Meeting the Challenges of Changing a Diet

Good nutrition is the goal, but food is not just about nutrition. It is about emotions, culture, and being social. What and how we eat is so personal that changing eating habits can be difficult. Special diets and drastic fitness programs sometimes promise the quick fix, or even the cure. Yet, the best advice for care receivers is the same as for everyone: Eat a low-fat and low-sodium diet with a variety of grains, vegetables, and fruits, along with some high-protein foods like meat or dairy products; and balance how many calories you take in with physical activity.

Deciding to change is the first step. But the changes don't have to take place overnight. Start with the easy ones. Then, one by one, add more kinds of vegetables, reduce portion sizes, start eating more low-fat foods.

Here's a checklist for you and the person in your care:

- Be realistic. Make small changes over time. Small steps can work better than giant leaps.

- Be daring and try new foods.

- Be flexible. Balance food intake with physical activity over several days. Don't focus on just one meal or one day.

- Be sensible and practice not overdoing it.

- Be active and choose activities that you enjoy and that fit into the rest of your life.

 Research shows that when individuals have confidence in their ability to do something, they are more likely to follow through, even under stressful conditions.

Special Needs and Considerations

Good nutrition is necessary for everyone, but sometimes things can get in the way of eating right. Ask the nurse, doctor, or pharmacist if any of the medications the person in your care is taking have possible side effects that can interfere with appetite or affect the absorption of important vitamins and minerals.

Here are some tips to ensure that the person in your care gets the nutrition he or she needs.

- The thought of three big meals may be too much for the person. In fact, five to six smaller mini-meals throughout the day may be easier to manage and help keep energy levels high. Keep the fridge and pantry filled with items that provide the nutrition the person in your care needs for good health and watch those that provide little to the diet except calories. Some healthful choices can include reduced-fat cheese sticks, nuts and nut butter, fresh or dried fruit, hardboiled eggs, low-fat yogurt or cottage cheese, bagged salads, and cut raw vegetables.

- Keep meal preparation simple. Focus on one part of the meal, like the main dish and rely on quick-cooking grains, easy-to-heat veggies and a whole-grain roll for side dishes. Save energy by collecting all the ingredients and cooking utensils first and sit down at the counter or table to put it all together.

- When you cook, try to make more than is needed for one meal. Store or freeze the rest in oven or microwave-ready containers for quick reheating.

- Make the most of the freezer. Stock up on low-salt dinners that can be quickly reheated.

- Save menus from places that deliver healthful meals.

Changes in mobility. If eating habits remain the same while activity drops off, **weight gain** can result. Added weight can increase fatigue, further limit mobility, put a strain on the respiratory and circulatory systems (lungs, heart, blood, blood vessels), and increase the risk of other chronic illnesses. Ask a registered dietitian to recommend an ideal weight and reasonable daily calorie intake to maintain that weight. To get weight under control, pair exercise with healthy eating.

Exercise for the person with heart failure can be challenging. There may be some days when his ability to exercise is limited. On those days, even sitting up in a chair and helping with daily grooming can be beneficial. As the caregiver, it is important to be patient on these "bad" days.

Eating and emotions. Depression can affect people's appetite in different ways. Many people turn to certain foods for comfort when they are depressed. These may be old favorites from childhood—a scoop of mashed potatoes, macaroni and cheese, a bowl of rice pudding. The danger is in overdoing it.

These foods are often high in fat, sugar, salt and calories that can easily add up. On the other hand, some people lose their appetite when they are depressed. Eating with others can help you and the person in your care stay connected. Physical movement and activity can help to improve mood and may also help spark appetite.

Bladder problems are another issue, most often created by the use of diuretics or "water pills" prescribed for people with heart failure. Often, fear of having to go to the bathroom frequently or loss of bladder control causes a person to limit fluids. This can cause other problems such as dehydration, dry mouth, difficulty swallowing, loss of appetite, and constipation. Find ways to fit in fluids. Here are some suggestions for how to do that:

- Take water breaks during the day.
- Have a beverage with meals.
- Take a drink when passing a water fountain.
- Travel with your own personal supply of bottled water.

NOTE A person with heart failure may find it hard to balance between dehydration and sticking to fluid restriction. This may take some getting used to, but over-drinking may cause an increase in symptoms for the person in your care. Speak to the doctor prior to consuming extra fluids.

Bowel management often involves preventing constipation. Fiber counts ... add it up. Fiber is found in cereal, grains, nuts, seeds, vegetables, and fruit. It is not completely digested (broken down) or absorbed (taken in) by the body. A diet rich in fiber (about 25 to 30 grams each day) along with recommended fluid intake and physical activity can help promote good bowel function. Fiber can also provide a sense of fullness, which helps in managing how much one eats.

Exercise as Part of Life

For the person with heart failure, nutrition and activity are a challenge. Even if physical activity is limited, moving a little each day is important. On a day when the person in your care feels better, she can be more active. It is not uncommon for a person with a cardiac condition to feel frightened about activity. However, it is still vital for her to participate in some sort of activity, even if it is simply bathing and dressing, so she doesn't think of herself as a "cardiac cripple."

Physical activity and good nutrition are perfect partners in good health. This winning combination finds a balance between what one eats and one's daily activities. Together, they help in managing weight and providing energy. Physical activity not only burns calories, but it can also help the person in your care by doing the following:

- Make the most of muscle strength, or even build strength, depending on the program.

- Slowly increase the ability to do more for longer periods of time.

- Increase range of motion and joint flexibility (the ability to move easily).

- Decrease feelings of fatigue.

- Decrease symptoms of depression.

- Maintain regular bowel and bladder functions.

- Cut down on the risk of skin breakdown and irritation.

- Protect weight-bearing bone mass (spine, hips, legs).

Good physical fitness is made up of three types of exercise: stretching, strengthening, and aerobics. Each is important by itself, but together they can help the person in your care remain active as long as possible. This will help the person deal better with the changes illness may bring.

A person should always stretch before exercise. This warms the muscles, helps prevent stiffness, and improves flexibility and balance. The person should work at his or her own pace, even if it seems very slow. Encourage the person in your care, even if the exercises seem difficult at first. Watch for signs of fatigue. Always cool down after exercise.

Stretching

Regular *s-t-r-e-t-c-h-i-n-g* is the first step, and it can be one of the most enjoyable. Stretching helps muscle rigidity (stiffness). It also helps muscles and joints stay flexible (able to bend). People who are more flexible have an easier time with everyday movement.

Stretching increases range of motion of joints and helps with good posture. It protects against muscle strains or sprains, improves circulation, and releases muscle tension.

Do's and Don'ts of Stretching

- **DO** stretch to the point of a gentle pull.

- **DON'T** stretch to the point of pain.

- **DON'T** bounce while stretching.

- **DON'T** hold the breath during a stretch. Breathe evenly in and out during each stretch.

- **DON'T** compare yourself to others.

Stretching can be done at any time. The person in your care can start the day by stretching before getting out of bed. Have the person stretch throughout the day.

Aerobic activities raise the heart rate and breathing, and promote cardiovascular (heart and lung) fitness. Even though people with heart failure have trouble exercising because of shortness of breath, slow-paced walking provides adequate aerobic exercise.

Some key points to remember:

- Regular exercise can help a person maintain mobility.

- You and the person in your care should talk with the doctor about exercise, target weight, and special needs. If possible, get a referral to a physical therapist or cardiac rehabilitation class to help begin the program.

- An exercise program needs to match the abilities and limitations of the individual. A physical therapist can design a well-balanced exercise program for those who need more help. With some changes, people at all levels of disability can enjoy the benefits of exercise.

- The person in your care should commit to doing what he can do on a consistent basis. Choosing activities you both enjoy will help you stick to your fitness plan. It may help to have a specific time set aside each day for activity.

- Start slowly. If the person in your care hasn't been active, begin at a low level of intensity for short periods. Alternate brief periods of exercise with periods of rest until the person in your care begins to build up endurance. Gradually increase activity and the length of time you are doing it.

- If the person in your care is able to get out of the house, she may be able to attend a group activity or exercise program in the community. Some local YMCA/YWCA's offer these programs.

Exercise and the Daily Routine

A good exercise regimen can help a person with heart failure feel better, decrease symptoms, and improve heart function. Some days the heart patient may not feel as well as other days. Even on those days, try to fit exercise and stretching into the daily routine.

- Find a simple activity that the person enjoys, such as walking, gardening, housekeeping, or swimming. As caregiver, you can try to make some of these activities part of the daily routine.

- Start very slowly and steadily increase the activity of the person in your care.

- Household chores such as folding laundry, dusting, wiping dishes, or helping with food preparation provide gentle exercise.

- Build a routine for scheduled activity, like taking a walk after breakfast or dinner.

- Music creates movement such as marching or dancing. If balance is a problem, try chair dancing. "Conducting" to the beat of up-tempo music provides upper body exercise and good emotional therapy!

- Perform a few extra arm and leg motions during dressing tasks.

A physical therapist can suggest exercises and stretches that will suit the person in your care. Therapists can also provide ways to improve walking and balance, if necessary.

Get Moving

In addition to a diet prescription, the person in your care may have gotten an exercise prescription. It is important that care receivers participate in some form of calorie-burning activity if at all possible.

For many disabled people, because of age or level of debility, the standard exercise prescription of 30 minutes most days of the week is simply not possible. So understand from the beginning that the activity level of the person in your care won't look like a healthy person's.

In Water

Water therapy is a time-tested form of healing. It is also a safe way for a person with a disability to exercise because there is no danger of falling. Floating in water allows easy movement and little strain on joints and muscles.

Using a kickboard or simply walking in place in water may produce aerobic benefit. Water also resists movement so it produces increased heart rate in less time. Water can also be a good place to exercise for those with balance problems. Talk to a physical therapist about whether a water aerobics class might be appropriate for the person in your care.

 Tip   YMCAs often offer water aerobics classes that the person in your care might participate in.

Fear of Falling

Balance can be affected in a person with a disability. If the person in your care has balance problems, dizziness, or a spinning sensation, see if you can get a physical therapy prescription from your doctor.

To reduce fear of falling, therapists often have people practice getting up from a lying position. This increases confidence that they can get up if they fall.

NOTE Persons with heart failure are usually on medication that can lower blood pressure and cause them to feel dizzy and lightheaded. Monitor blood pressure at home and notify the doctor if low blood pressure readings are persistent. The doctor may need to adjust medications to help improve blood pressure readings and decrease feelings of dizziness.

Remember, before starting any type of workout routine, get advice from your physician. Start slowly with only moderate effort. Give the care receiver time to build strength and stamina. Any amount of exercise helps reduce risk, and the benefits of exercise are cumulative, so find a way to make it easy to get exercise, that way the care receiver is more likely to do it. Exercise is a particularly effective way to reduce depression.

And finally, everything said here about the benefits of aerobic exercise and weight training also applies to the caregiver. *You* need exercise as much as the person in your care. Find a way to make it part of most days. (See Chapter 11, *How to Avoid Caregiver Burnout*)

Driving

There are no set rules or limitations concerning people with heart failure driving a car. As a caregiver, factors that you should consider are whether or not the person in your care has physical or mental changes that decrease his ability to drive. Some of these changes may include confusion, excessive fatigue, or memory lapses. If you are unsure, discuss your concerns with your health care team.

Motivation

Motivation is the #1 factor determining whether people change their lifestyles or fail to follow their exercise and diet prescriptions. While the person in your care needs to be motivated, the caregiver has a part to play, too. Do what you can to make exercise fun. Make the new diet an experiment. If you make either diet or exercise too important, any failure becomes that much more significant. Keep it light hearted, maintain a sense of humor, and join in as much as possible.

No single day of exercise or eating right makes much of a difference in a person's health, but 30 days do. Sixty days makes even more of an impact; a year's worth of a new lifestyle can provide changes in mood, independence and self-esteem.

NOTE Even though exercise and motivation are important in daily routine of the person in your care, it is equally important for you, the caregiver. Remember, that taking even 10 –"take care of yourself moments" a day helps ensure your health.

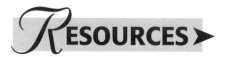

American Dietetic Association
www.eatright.org
(800) 366-1655
Call weekdays 10:00 a.m. to 5:00 p.m. EST to locate a registered dietitian in your area.

Area Agency on Aging or the Cooperative Extension Service
Your local office offers free counseling by a registered dietitian.

Meals-on-Wheels

Can provide nutritious meals delivered to the home. Check with your local Department of Aging or your Community Department of Human Services.

MyPyramid

www.mypyramid.gov

This replaces the old Food Guide Pyramid. It is a very interactive site to help people make healthy choices consistent with the latest Dietary Guidelines for Americans.

The National Sports Center for the Disabled (NSCD)

P.O. Box 1290

Winter Park, CO 80482

(970) 726-1540

www.nscd.org

E-mail: info@nscd.org

NSCD is a nonprofit corporation that offers winter and summer recreation. Winter sports include snow skiing, snowshoeing, and cross-country skiing. Summer recreation activities include fishing, hiking, rock climbing, whitewater rafting, camping, mountain biking, sailing, therapeutic horseback riding, and a baseball camp.

American Heart Association

7272 Greenville Avenue

Dallas, TX 75231

Phone: (214) 373-6300 or

1-800-AHA-USA1

www.amhrt.org

The American Association of Cardiovascular and Pulmonary Rehabilitation (AACVPR)

http://www.aacvpr.org/certification/program_cert_search.cfm

Offers a list of available cardiac rehabilitation programs in all states.

Heart Failure Society of America, Inc.
Box 358
420 Delaware Street, SE
Minneapolis, MN 55455
Phone: (612) 626-3864
www.hfsa.org

The Alliance for Aging Research
2021 K Street, NW
Suite 305
Washington, DC 20006
Phone: (202)293-2856
www.agingresearch.org

Publication

A Modification of the Rules of Golf for Golfers with Disabilities

United States Golf Association
P.O. Box 708
Far Hills, NJ 07931-0708
(908) 234-2300
www.usga.org/playing/rules/golfers_with_disabilities.html
Online publication contains permissible modifications to the rules of golf for players with a disability.

If you don't have access to the Internet, ask your local library to help you locate a Web site.

Emergencies

Emergencies

*E*mergency situations are common when caring for a person with chronic illness. Many injuries can be avoided through preventive measures. (📖 *See Chapter 12,* **Activities of Daily Living**). When a crisis does occur, use common sense, stay calm, and realize that you can help.

> **NOTE** ▶ Make sure 911 is posted on your phone or ideally is on speed-dial. Keep written driving instructions near the phone for how to get to your house. If you have a speakerphone, use the speaker when talking to the dispatcher. This way, you can follow the dispatcher's instructions while attending to the emergency.

When to Call for an Ambulance

Call for an ambulance if a person—

- has fainted, passed out, or becomes unconscious
- has chest pain, pressure, or discomfort that lasts for more than a few minutes or if it is NOT relieved with rest or nitroglycerin
- has severe, persistent shortness of breath
- has no signs of breathing (no movement or response to touch or voice)
- is bleeding severely
- is vomiting blood or is bleeding from the rectum
- has fallen and may have broken bones

- has had a seizure

- has a severe headache and slurred speech

- has pressure or severe pain in the abdomen that does not go away

OR

- if moving the person could cause further injury

- if traffic or distance would cause a life-threatening delay in getting to the hospital

- if the person is too heavy for you to lift or help

Ambulance service is expensive and may not be covered by insurance. Use it when you believe there is an emergency.

In an emergency:

Step 1: Call 911.
Step 2: Care for the victim.

Also call 911 for emergencies involving fire, explosion, poisonous gas, fallen electrical wires, or other life-threatening situations.

 If the person in your care has signed a Do Not Resuscitate (DNR) order, have it available to show the paramedics. Otherwise, they are required to initiate resuscitation (reviving the person). The order must go with the patient. The Do Not Resuscitate order must be with the patient at all times.

In the Emergency Room

Be sure you understand the instructions for care *before* leaving the emergency room. Call the patient's personal doctor as soon as possible and let him or her know about the emergency room care.

Bring to the emergency room—

- insurance policy numbers

- a list of medical problems

- a list of medications currently being taken

- the personal physician's name and phone number

- the name and number of a relative or friend of the person in your care

NOTE You may want to keep a copy of all of the above information in an envelope. Make sure it is located in an easy-to-remember and easy-to-reach location. We strongly suggest that you take a course in CPR from your local American Red Cross, hospital, or other agency.

Choking (Adult)

Prevention

- Avoid serving alcohol.

- Make sure the person in your care has a good set of dentures to chew food properly.

- Cut the food into small pieces.

- Do not encourage the person to talk while eating.

- Do not make the person laugh while eating.

- Learn the Heimlich maneuver in CPR class.

Bleeding

If someone is bleeding heavily, protect yourself with rubber gloves, plastic wrap, or layers of cloth. Then—

1. Apply direct pressure over the wound with a clean cloth.

2. Apply another clean cloth on top of the blood-soaked cloth, keeping the pressure firm.

3. If no bones are broken, elevate (raise) the injured limb to decrease blood flow.

4. Call 911 for an ambulance.

5. Apply a bandage snugly over the dressing.

6. Wash your hands with soap and water as soon as possible after providing care.

7. Avoid contact with blood-soaked objects.

Shock

Shock may be associated with heavy bleeding, hives, shortness of breath, dizziness, swelling, thirst, and chest pain. The signs of shock are:

- restlessness and irritability

- confusion, altered consciousness

- pale, cool, moist skin

- rapid breathing and weakness

If these signs are present—

1. Have the person lie down.

2. Control any bleeding.

3. Keep the person warm.

4. Elevate the legs about 12 to 14 inches unless the neck or back has been injured.

5. Do not give the person anything to eat or drink.

6. Call 911.

Chest Pain

Any chest pain that lasts more than a few minutes is related to the heart until proven otherwise. CALL 911 IMMEDIATELY. Don't wait to see if it goes away. Danger signs include—

- pain radiating from the chest down the arms, up the neck to the jaw, and into the back

- crushing, squeezing chest pain or heavy pressure in the chest

- shortness of breath, sweating, nausea and vomiting, weakness

- bluish, pale skin

- skin that is moist

- excessive perspiration

If the person is unresponsive (no movement or response to touch or voice), **call 911.** Be prepared to give Rescue Breathing and start CPR as instructed in CPR class.

Falls and Related Injuries

Preventive measures include—

- staying in when it is rainy or icy outside

- having regular vision screening check-ups for correct eyeglasses

- using separate reading glasses and other regular glasses if bifocals make it difficult to see the floor

- being cautious when walking on wet floors

- wearing good foot support when walking

- being aware that new shoes are slippery and crepe-soled shoes can cause the toe to catch

- having foot pain problems corrected

- keeping toenails trimmed and feet healthy for good balance

Fainting

Fainting can be caused by—

- a heart attack

- medications

- low blood sugar

- standing up quickly

- straining to have a bowel movement

- dehydration

- a change in blood pressure

To some extent, fainting can be prevented.

- Ask the doctor if medications that do not cause fainting can be prescribed.

- Monitor blood sugar levels.

- Monitor blood pressure.

- Avoid constipation.

- Do not let the person stand up or sit up too rapidly.

Monitor blood pressure readings if the person in your care is on medications that can lower her blood pressure and cannot be discontinued. If systolic blood pressure (the top number) is lower than 85, contact the doctor. He may want to lower the dose of certain medications to prevent these low blood pressure readings. By doing this, the person's "dizziness" may improve. But remember, you or the person in your care should NEVER change medications without the doctor's advice.

If a fainting spell occurs:

1. Do not try to place the person in a sitting position. Instead, immediately lay him down flat.

2. Check the person's airway, breathing, and pulse.

3. Turn the person on his side.

4. Elevate the legs.

5. Cover him with a blanket if the room or floor is cold.

6. Do not give fluids.

7. Call 911 if person is having difficulty breathing, not breathing, or not responding to your voice and touch.

8. If not breathing, be prepared to give Rescue Breathing and start CPR as instructed in CPR class.

Heat Stroke

Some medications can increase the likelihood of heat stroke. To prevent heat stroke—

• Ask the doctor if the medicine the person is taking can increase the risk of heat stroke.

- Use clothing made of breathable lightweight fabrics.

- Use a fan, damp compresses, or an air conditioner.

- Have the person continue to drink fluids per their daily fluid restriction. Remember, a glass of ice chips lasts longer and is equivalent to only half a glass of water once melted.

- Avoid alcohol, caffeine, and smoking because they speed dehydration.

- Avoid activity during the hottest part of the day.

Signs of heat stroke include headache, nausea, and sudden dizziness. Consult the doctor immediately to determine whether it is a serious condition. Call 911 if you suspect heat stroke.

Stroke

Strokes occur when the blood flow to the brain is interrupted by a clogged or burst blood vessel. Strokes cannot always be prevented, but the chances of their occurring can be lessened through—

- a balanced diet

- avoidance of stress

- periodic checkups

- regular exercise

- regular blood pressure monitoring

- regular use of a prescribed blood pressure medicine

Suspect a stroke when the person in your care—

- has a sudden and severe headache

- does not respond to simple statements

- has a seizure

- is suddenly incontinent (unable to control bladder and bowel)

- has paralysis (cannot move) in an arm or leg

- cannot grip equally with both hands

- appears droopy on one side of the face

- has slurred speech or blurred vision

- is confused

- has an unsteady gait

- has trouble swallowing

- has loss of balance or coordination when combined with one of the other signs

The chance of recovery from a stroke is greatly increased if the person has immediate help.

1. Keep the person in the position you found him in.

2. Reassure him and keep him calm.

3. If he has trouble breathing, open his airway, tilt his head, and lift his chin.

4. Call 911. Get the person to medical care as soon as possible.

5. If the person is not breathing, give 2 Rescue Breaths.

6. If breathing resumes, place the person on one side to prevent choking. This also helps keep the tongue out of the airway.

7. If the person is unresponsive (no movement or response to touch or voice), be prepared to give Rescue Breathing and start CPR as instructed in CPR class.

Checklist **Home First Aid Kit**

Buy or make a home first-aid kit. Note on the box the date when the item was purchased. Check and replenish your supplies at least once a year. These should include the following:

✓ *antibiotic ointment*

✓ *Band-Aids®*

✓ *disinfectant for cleaning wounds*

✓ *disposable gloves*

✓ *emergency telephone numbers*

✓ *eye pads*

✓ *instant ice packs*

✓ *list of current medications*

✓ *pocket mask/face mask*

✓ *rolled gauze and elastic bandages*

✓ *scissors*

✓ *sterile gauze bandages (nonstick 4 × 4)*

✓ *syrup of ipecac*

✓ *thermometer*

✓ *tongue depressors*

✓ *3-ounce rubber bulb to rinse out wounds*

✓ *triangle bandage*

✓ *tweezers and needle*

Hospice Care

Hospice Care

Preparing for Hospice Care

Addressing end-of-life issues is difficult for most people. However, this life stage can give the person who is terminally ill and her family the time to examine life, establish priorities, and renew or strengthen relationships. During this time, you can help in easing the transition by participating in choices in hospice care. A hospice team can help ensure that the person in your care is as comfortable as possible during this period. It can also guide the patient's and family's choices for final arrangements.

When an Illness Takes a Turn for the Worse

When a serious illness becomes life threatening, a person will go through many physical, emotional, and spiritual changes. Decisions to end medical treatment, seek hospice care, or to withdraw life support may need to be made. It's best to talk over these decisions with the physicians and family of the person in your care well before there is a health care crisis.

Discussing the Person's Wishes

- When possible, discuss the person's and the family's wishes before an illness reaches the final phase.

- Does the person have a health care proxy?

- Is there a living will or medical power of attorney?

- What would the person's choices be regarding life support?

- Would the person want to stay at home or enter a facility?

The Principles of Hospice Care

Hospice has always recognized the importance of including the ill person, the family, and other loved ones in the care plan. Caregiving for someone who is dying can be demanding and it's important for everyone involved with a terminal illness to take proper care of his needs.

Hospice services can provide expert, compassionate care and make it possible for a dying person to remain at home. The earlier hospice care begins, the more it can help in providing the care needed at this time. It can also help loved ones enjoy the best quality of life as a family unit. The focus of hospice is on care, not cure.

Questions to Ask When Choosing a Program

There are more than 3,100 hospices in this country and the hospice in your community can provide information and help you answer some of the difficult decisions that accompany terminal illness and dying. Here are some questions you can ask in selecting hospice care:

- Is the agency licensed and accredited by a nationally recognized organization?

- Are they Medicare certified?

- What are their billing policies and payment plans?

- Can they provide references, such as local hospital and care centers, institutions, and caregivers?

- How do they decide whether an individual is ready for hospice care?

- How are their caregivers supervised?

- What are their expectations about the family's sharing in caregiving?

- Are you comfortable with the program? Does it feel like the right fit?

What Hospice Care Provides

Hospice is a concept of medical care that delivers comfort and support to people in the final stages of a terminal illness and to their families. Care is delivered by a team of specially trained medical professionals who focus on easing pain and managing symptoms. They provide medical, emotional, psychological, and spiritual care to the person and family. They assist the family in coping with their coming loss and their grief afterward.

Most hospice care is delivered in the home, but hospice care can also be provided in nursing homes and hospice facilities. The person who is ill and the family are the core of the hospice team and are at the center of all decision making.

Although a family member or other caregiver cares for the person on a daily basis, a hospice nurse is available 24 hours a day to provide advice and make visits. Hospice services include

- physician services

- nursing services

- medical social services

- home health aide and homemaker services

- spiritual, dietary, and other counseling

- physical, occupational, and speech–language therapy

- medicine for controlling pain

- medical supplies and appliances

- ongoing care at home during periods of crisis

- special services for grief counseling

- trained volunteers for companionship, errands, or respite

- short-term inpatient care

- bereavement (grief) services for the family (or loved ones) for up to a year after death

Although the attending physician typically refers a person to hospice, a family member, friend, or caregiver may also make the referral to hospice. The hospice nurse will contact the doctor for an order for care if that is the wish of the terminally ill person. Any terminal disease or illness qualifies.

Criteria for Admission to a Hospice Care Program

To qualify for hospice care, this condition must be met:

The person must be certified as terminally ill by his or her doctor and the hospice medical director. "Terminally ill" means having a life expectancy of six months or less if the disease runs its normal course.

To qualify for Medicare coverage of hospice a person must meet the following four conditions:

- The patient is eligible for Medicare part A

- The patient's doctor and the hospice medical director certify that the patient is terminally ill with six months or less to live if the disease runs its expected course.

- The patient signs a statement choosing hospice care instead of standard Medicare benefits for the terminal illness.

- The patient receives care from a Medicare-approved hospice program.

Hospice care is offered for two periods of 90 days, followed by an unlimited number of 60-day periods, as long as the physician recertifies that the patient is not getting better and is still terminal. The hospice team will assess for signs of decline or worsening. A patient may leave hospice care if his or her condition improves, and reenter if the condition worsens.

How to Pay for Hospice Care

Hospice care is a benefit under Medicare Hospital Insurance (Part A) to beneficiaries with a very limited life expectancy. To receive Medicare payments, the agency or organization must be approved by Medicare to provide hospice services. Under Medicare, hospice is primarily a program of care delivered in the person's home by a Medicare-approved hospice to provide comfort and relief from pain.

The out-of-pocket expense for the patient is a 5 percent copayment for patient respite care and prescription drugs (not to exceed $5 for prescriptions). There are no deductibles under the Medicare hospice program.

When all requirements are met, Medicare covers:

- doctor services
- nursing care
- medical appliances
- medical supplies
- drugs for symptom management and pain relief
- home health aide and homemaker services
- physical and occupational therapy
- speech/language pathology services
- medical social service
- dietary and counseling services
- psychological counseling for emotional support to patient and family
- spiritual counseling to patient and family
- respite services for the family
- volunteer assistance for companionship and respite

What Medicare will not cover:

- Treatment intended to cure your medical illness.

- Prescriptions to cure your illness rather than symptom control or pain relief. (Medications unrelated to the terminal illness will be covered.)

- Medical care from a provider other than the hospice team.

- Care in an emergency room or inpatient facility is not covered unless it was arranged by your hospice medical team.

Respite Care

Respite care is provided to the hospice patient by another caregiver so that the primary caregiver can have a rest or a change in routine. Sometimes the caregiver may need someone else to provide care so that they can have a break from day-to-day responsibilities. Also, the caregiver may need assistance if an emergency develops for her and she must attend to other matters. This is usually for a short period of time. During respite care, the person being cared for will be taken care of at a Medicare-approved facility, such as a hospice inpatient facility, hospital or skilled nursing facility. As a caregiver, you may be reluctant to think about respite care, but as we have emphasized throughout the book, you must take care of yourself, and you can't handle all the responsibilities of providing care by yourself. Respite care is a Medicare-approved benefit.

> **NOTE** Hospice care as a Medicare benefit can be received for two 90-day periods followed by an unlimited number of 60-day periods. The physician must recertify the person's terminal condition at the beginning of each period. Hospice is also covered under Medicaid in 41 states and by most insurance plans and HMOs.

The Experience of Grief

Grieving is a natural and important process that helps us avoid depression and psychological problems later. The stages of grief are different for all of us—and the time it takes to pass through them varies. (In general, one must experience at least one set of seasons and holidays without a loved one, but often the grieving process takes much longer than that.)

As you grieve, you may experience intense and conflicting emotions and you may feel at times that you are not in control of these reactions. This happens to many people. However, by recognizing the common stages of grief, you can handle feelings that might otherwise be alarming. Remember, the grieving process is natural and, ultimately, will restore balance to your life.

These are some common stages in the grieving process:

- shock and numbness—usually the first stage, which can last from a few days to several months

- denial—a refusal to accept the loss

- realization and emotional release—feelings of overwhelming sadness and bouts of crying, often at unexpected times

- guilt—feelings that more could have been done

- disorganization and anxiety—confusion and an inability to concentrate, causing feelings of panic

- memory flashbacks—sudden flashbacks of both good and bad memories

- loneliness and depression—a long period of overwhelming sadness and loss of interest in things that once gave pleasure

- anger and resentment—at the doctors, the family, friends, God, and even the person who died

- recovery and acceptance—a return to a more normal life

 It is helpful to deal with grief by being around people who have gone through the same experience. Most communities have grief support groups through churches, synagogues, county mental health departments, and other nonprofit organizations. Hospice programs also offer support groups for survivors.

Serious Warning Signs

Seek professional counseling if you or a family member develops a medical condition in reaction to profound feelings of loss or:

- feels strong hostility

- loses all emotional feeling

- begins using alcohol or drugs

- feels happiness instead of a sense of loss

- withdraws from all friendships

- is profoundly depressed

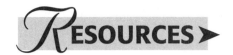

RESOURCES ➤

Hospice Foundation of America
2001 S Street NW, #300
Washington, DC 20009
Tel: (800) 854-3402
www.hospicefoundation.org
Provides information and referral service, resources on end-of-life care, a search engine to end-of-life Web sites, free brochures on hospice, volunteering, and bereavement.

National Hospice and Palliative Care Organization
Tel: Hotline (800) 658-8898; (703) 243-5900
www.nhpco.org
Provides information on hospice, referrals to local hospices, and outreach hospice services to families of dying people.

U. S. Department of Health & Human Services
Centers for Medicare and Medicaid
"Medicare Hospice Benefits"
www.medicare.gov

Respite Services

ARCH National Respite Locator Service
800 Eastowne Drive, Suite 105
Chapel Hill, NC 27514-2204
(919) 490-5577
www.respitelocator.org
Provides caregivers with contact information on respite services in their area.

Call your local **Social Security Administration, State Health Department, State Hospice Organization,** or call (800) 633-4227 **Medicare Hotline** to learn about hospice benefits.

If you don't have home access to the Internet, ask your local library to help you locate any Web site.

Part Three: Additional Resources

Common Abbreviations

MI – heart attack

ADA – Americans with Disabilities Act

ADL – activities of daily living

ASHD – arteriosclerotic heart disease

BC – blood culture

BID – 2 times per day (approximately 8 and 8 as medication times)

BP – blood pressure

BRP – bathroom privileges

BS – blood sugar

C&S – culture and sensitivity

CA – cancer/carcinoma

CABG – coronary artery bypass graft

CBC – complete blood count

CCU – coronary care unit

CHF – congestive heart failure

CHIRP – Cardiac Health Improvement and Rehabilitation Program

CNS – central nervous system

COPD – chronic obstructive pulmonary disease

CPR – cardiopulmonary resuscitation

CTS – cardiothoracic surgery

CVA – cerebral vascular accident

DM – diabetes mellitus

DME – durable medical equipment

DNR – do not resuscitate

DRG – diagnosis related group

Dx – diagnosis

ECF – extended care facility

ED – emergency department

EEG – electroencephalogram recording of the brain's electrical activity

EKG/ECG – electrocardiogram recording of the heart's electrical activity

EP – electrophysiology

FBS – fasting blood sugar, or the amount of glucose in the blood when a person has not eaten for 12 hours

FX – fracture

GTT – glucose tolerance test to determine a person's ability to metabolize glucose

HC – home care

HHA – a home health agency providing home health services

HS – hour of sleep (medication time)

I&O – record of food and liquid taken in and waste eliminated

ICU – intensive care unit for special monitoring of the acutely ill

IV – intravenous line to drip fluids and blood products into the bloodstream

LOC – loss of consciousness

LVAD – Left ventricular assist device

MCD – Medicaid

MCR – Medicare

MRI – magnetic resonance imaging

Neuro – neurologist

NPO – nothing by mouth

NP – Nurse practitioner

NSAID – nonsteroid antiinflammatory drug.

OR – operating room

OT – occupational therapy or occupational therapist

PO – by mouth

Psych – psychologist

PT – physical therapy or physical therapist

QID – 4 times per day (approximately 9–1–5–9 as medication times)

RBC – red blood count

RN – nurse

ROM – range of motion

RR – respiratory rate

RVAD – right ventricular assist device

Rx – prescription

SNF – skilled nursing facility

SOB – shortness of breath

SS or SSA – Social Security or Social Security Administration

SSI/SSD – supplemental security income or diability income

ST – Speech therapist or speech therapy

Sx – symptoms

TIA – transient ischemic attack

TID – 3 times per day (approximately 9–1–6 as medication times)

TPR – temperature, pulse, respiration

TX – treatment

U/A – urine analysis

VNS – visiting nurse service

WBC – white blood count

Common Specialists

Anesthesiologist
Pain relief during and after surgery

Cardiac Health Improvement and Rehabilitation Program (CHIRP)
A cardiac rehabilitation program is designed to help the person in your care exercise safely and maintain a heart-healthy lifestyle.

Cardiologist
Conditions of the heart, lungs, and blood vessels

Dietitian
A registered dietitian can provide in-depth personalized nutrition education and help you help the person in your care begin a personal action plan.

Dentist
Teeth and gums

Dermatologist
Skin, hair, and nails

Electrophysiologist
A cardiologist who specializes in diagnosing and treating irregular heart rhythms caused by problems with the heart's electrical system.

Endocrinologist
Hormonal problems including thyroid disorders

Gastroenterologist
Digestive system, stomach, liver bowels, and gallbladder

Geriatrician
Disorders common to elderly persons

Hematologist
Diseases of the blood, spleen, and lymph glands

Internist
Primary care of common illnesses, both long term and emergency

Nephrologist
Kidney diseases and disorders

Neurologist
Brain and nervous system disorders

Nurse Practitioner
Provides preventive and medical health care in association with a physician

Oncologist
All cancers

Ophthalmologist
Care and surgery of the eyes

Optician
Fitting and making of eyeglasses and contact lenses

Optometrist
Basic eye care

Oral Maxillofacial Surgeon
Surgery involving the teeth, gums, and jaw

Orthopedist
Surgery involving joints, bones, and muscles

Otolaryngologist
Head and neck surgeon

Occupational Therapist
An occupational therapist specializes in helping people to reach their maximum level of function and independence in all aspects of daily life.

Pharmacist
Medications specialist; provider of physician and patient education

Physical Therapist
A health care professional who teaches exercises and physical activities that help condition muscles and restore strength and movement safely, while increasing stamina.

Podiatrist
Foot care

Psychiatrist (MD)
Emotional, mental, or addictive disorders

Psychologist (MA or PhD)
Assessment and care of emotional or mental disorders

Pulmonologist
Diseases of lungs and airways

Rheumatologist
Diseases of joints and connective tissue (arthritis)

Surgeon and/or Transplant Surgeon
A specialist who operates on the heart, including implanting ventricular assist devices (VAD) and heart transplants.

Urologist
Urinary system and the male reproductive system

Caregiver Organizations

Caregiver Information and Support Organizations

. . . And Thou Shalt Honor

http://www.thoushalthonor.org/

The site for the acclaimed PBS caregiving documentary . . . And Thou Shalt Honor provides a variety of caregiving tools and resources.

Everyday Warriors

www.everydaywarriors.com

This site features numerous articles of interest to caregivers of all ages. Visit "Ask the Caregiver Coach," and "Caregivers Sound Off."

FamilyCare America, Inc.

1004 N. Thompson St., Suite 205
Richmond, VA 23230
(804) 342-2200
www.FamilyCareAmerica.com

FamilyCare America is dedicated to improving the lives of caregivers of the elderly, disabled, and chronically ill by creating a highly accessible resource where caregivers can:

- *better learn the process of caregiving*
- *receive help in managing their fears and concerns*
- *obtain resources for help with all aspects of caregiving*

267

Family Caregivers Alliance
690 Market Street, Suite 600
San Francisco, CA 94104
(800) 445-8106; 415-434-3388 Fax: (415) 434-3508
www.caregiver.org
E-mail: info@caregiver.org
Resource center for caregivers of people with chronic disabling conditions. The Web site provides information on services and programs in education, research, and advocacy.

National Alliance for Caregiving
4720 Montgomery Lane, 5th Floor
Bethesda, MD 20814
www.caregiving.org
The Alliance is a non-profit coalition of national organizations focusing on issues of family caregiving.

National Family Caregivers Association
10400 Connecticut Avenue, Suite 500
Kensington, MD 20895
(800) 896-3650
www.thefamilycaregiver.org
The Association supports, empowers, educates, and speaks up for the more than 50 million Americans who care for a chronically ill, aged, or disabled person.

Well Spouse Association
63 West Main Street—Suite H
Freehold, NJ 07728
(800) 838-0879
www.wellspouse.org
E-mail: info@wellspouse.org
A national, not-for-profit membership organization that gives support to wives, husbands, and partners of the chronically ill and/or disabled.

Glossary

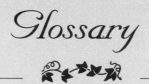

A

Activities of daily living (ADL): personal hygiene, bathing, dressing, grooming, toileting, feeding, and transferring

Acute: state of illness that comes on suddenly and may be of short duration

Advance directive: a legal document that states a person's health care preferences in writing while that person is competent and able to make such decisions

Ambulatory: able to walk with little or no assistance

Analgesics: medications used to relieve pain

Antibiotics: a group of drugs used to combat infection

Apathy: a condition in which the person shows little or no emotion

Artificial life-support systems: the use of respirators, tube feeding, intravenous (IV) feeding, and other means to replace natural and vital functions, such as breathing, eating, and drinking

Assessment: the process of analyzing a person's condition

Assistive devices: any tools that are designed, fabricated, and/or adapted to assist a person in performing a particular task, e.g., cane, walker, show chair

Atrophy: the wasting away of muscles or brain tissue

B

Blood pressure: the pressure of the blood on the walls of the blood vessels and arteries

Body mechanics: proper use and positioning of the body to do work and avoid strain and injury

C

Calorie: the measure of the energy the body gets from various foods

CHIRP: helps your care receiver exercise safely and maintain a heart-healthy lifestyle

Chronic: refers to a state or condition that lasts 6 months or longer

Cognition: high-level functions carried out by the human brain, including comprehension and use of speech, visual perception and construction, calculation ability, attention (information processing), memory, and executive functions such as planning, problem-solving, and self-monitoring

Constipation: difficulty having bowel movements

D

Dietitian: person who can provide in-depth personalized nutrition education and help you begin your personal action plan.

Decubitus ulcer: pressure sore; bedsore

Defibrillator: a device that uses an electrical current to restore or regulate a stopped or disorganized heartbeat

Dehydration: loss of normal body fluid, sometimes caused by vomiting and severe diarrhea

Dementia: a progressive decline in mental functions

Depression: a psychiatric condition that can be moderate or severe and cause feelings of sadness and emptiness

Diuretics: drugs that help the body get rid of fluids

Durable Power of Attorney: a legal document that authorizes another to act as one's agent and is "durable" because it remains in effect in case the person becomes disabled or mentally incompetent

Durable Power of Attorney for Health Care Decisions: a legal document that lets a person name someone else to make health care decisions after the person has become disabled or mentally incompetent and is unable to make those decisions

E

Edema: an abnormal swelling in legs, ankles, hands, or abdomen that occurs because the body is retaining fluids

Estate planning: a process of planning for the present and future use of a person's assets

❧ F

Foot drop: a condition of weakness in the muscles of the foot and ankle, caused by poor nerve conduction, which interferes with a person's ability to flex the ankle and walk with a normal heel–toe pattern; the toes touch the ground before the heel, causing the person to trip or lose balance

❧ G

Gait: the manner in which a person walks
Geriatric: refers to people 65 or older
Guardian: the one who is designated to have protective care of another person or of that person's property

❧ H

Heimlich maneuver: a method for clearing the airway of a choking person
Hospice: a program that allows a dying person to remain at home while receiving professionally supervised care

❧ I

Incontinence: involuntary discharge of urine or feces
Intravenous (IV): the delivery of fluids, medications, or nutrients into a vein

❧ L

Laxative: a substance taken to increase bowel movements and prevent constipation

❧ M

Medic-Alert®: bracelet identification system linked to a 24-hour service that provides full information in the case of an emergency

Medicaid: a public health program that uses state and federal funds to pay certain medical and hospital expenses of those having low income or no income, with benefits that vary from state to state

Medicare: the federal health insurance program for people 65 or older and for certain people under 65 who are disabled

✲ N

Nutrition: a process of giving the body the key nutrients it needs for proper body function

✲ O

Occupational therapy: therapy that focuses on the activities of daily living such as personal hygiene, bathing, dressing, grooming, toileting, and feeding

Ombudsman: a person who helps residents of a retirement or health care facility with such problems as quality of care, food, finances, medical care, residents rights, and other concerns; these services are confidential and free

Oral hygiene: the process of keeping the mouth clean

✲ P

Paralysis: loss or impairment of voluntary movement of a group of muscles

Physical therapy: the process of relearning walking, balancing, and transfers

Positioning: placing a person in a position that allows functional activity and minimizes the danger of faulty posture that could cause pressure sores, impaired breathing, and shrinking of muscles and tendons

Power of Attorney for Health Care: providing another person with the authority to make health care decisions

Pressure sore: a breakdown of the skin caused by prolonged pressure in one spot; a bed sore; decubitus ulcer

Prognosis: a forecast of what is likely to happen when an individual contracts a particular disease or condition

✲ R

Range of motion (ROM): the extent of possible passive (movement by another person) movement in a joint

Rehabilitation: after a disabling injury or disease, restoration of a person's maximum physical, mental, vocational, social, and spiritual potential

Respite care: short-term care that allows a primary caregiver time off from his or her responsibilities

Rigidity: a tightness or increase in muscle tone at rest or throughout the entire range of motion of a limb, which may be felt as a stiffness by the patient

☙ S

Sedatives: medications used to calm a person

Shock: a state of collapse resulting from reduced blood volume and/or blood pressure caused by burns, severe injury, pain, or an emotional blow

Stroke: sudden loss of function of a part of the brain due to interference in its blood supply, usually by hemorrhage or blood clotting

Support groups: groups of people who get together to share common experiences and help one another cope

Symptom: sign of a disease or disorder that helps in diagnosis

☙ T

Transfer: movements from one position to another, for example, from bed to chair, wheelchair to car, etc.

Transfer belt: a device placed around the waist of a disabled person and used to secure the person while walking; gait belt

☙ U

Urinal: a container used by a bedridden male for urinating

Urinalysis: a laboratory test of urine

☙ V

Vital signs: life signs such as blood pressure, breathing, and pulse

Void: to urinate; pass water

☙ W

Will: a legal document that states how to dispose of a person's property after death according to that person's wishes

Index

outside activities and, 158–159
respite time/respite zones and, 155–157
self-care for caregivers and, 151–154
stress relief and, 157–158

B-type natriuretic peptide (BNP), 27, 28
Basin bath, 166
Bathing
    basin bath in, 166
    bed bath in, 164–165
    showers and, 166
    tub baths in, 166
Bed bath, 164–165
Beta blockers, 41
Betapace. *See* Sotalol
Biofeedback, 201
Bisoprolol (Zebeta), 41
BIV. *See* biventricular pacemaker
Biventricular pacemaker (BIV), 45–46
Bladder management and diet, 227
Bleeding, 241
Blood pressure, 9–11, 17, 20, 222–223
    DASH Diet and, 222
    fainting and, 243–244
    falls and, fluctuations in, 233
    nutrition, diet and, 222–223
    salt/sodium restriction and, 222
    systolic and diastolic numbers in, 10–11, 10
Blood tests, 27–28
Boredom, 197–198
Bowel function and constipation, 175, 227
Breathing and pain management, 202
Bumetanide (Bumex), 42
Burnout. *See* avoiding caregiver burnout

C-reactive protein (CRP), 27
CABG. *See* coronary artery bypass graft
Calcium, 215–217
Calories, 152, 213–214, 219
Cancer treatments and heart failure, 12
Candesartan (Atacand), 41
Captopril (Capoten), 40
Cardiac catheterization, 29
Cardiac Health Improvement and Rehabilitation
        Program (CHIRP), 47, 265

Cardiac resynchronization therapy (CRT), 46
Cardiologist, 71, 265
Cardiomyopathy and heart failure, 12
Carvediol (Coreg), 41
Case management, 87–88
Catheterization, cardiac, 29
Causes of heart failure, 9–12
Center for Medicare/Medicaid Services
        (CMS), 110
Certified nurses aide (CNA), 98
Chambers of the heart, 7
Changes to report to the doctor, 76–77
Chest pain, 242
Chest x-rays, 28
Choking, 240
Cholesterol, 18, 21, 27, 220–221
Chronic pain management, 201
Cleaning techniques for infection control, 177
Clinic, 71
Clothing, 171
Cocaine and heart failure, 12
Commode use, 172
Communication, 194, 203
Community meals, 181
Community-based services, 118–119
Complementary medicine, 82
Compliance with treatment, 44
Computer activities, 198–199
Congenital heart defects and heart failure, 12
Congestive heart failure, 6
Constipation, 175
Continuing-care retirement communities, 61
Continuing education, 198
Contracts, housing options, 62, 64
Controllable risk factors, 16–18
Cordarone. *See* Amiodarone
Coreg. *See* Carvediol
Coronary angiography, 29
Coronary artery bypass graft (CABG), 45
Coronary artery disease, 9, 10, 16
Coumadin (Warfarin), 42
Cozaar. *See* Losartan
CRT. *See* cardiac resynchronization therapy
Crystodigin. *See* digoxin (digitalis)
Custodial care, 61

Oral/dental care, 83, 168–169
  dentures and, 168
Orthopedist, 266
Osteoporosis prevention, 215–216
Otolaryngologist, 266
Outside activities and caregiver burnout,
    158–159
Outside help for home care, 56, 58

Pacemakers in, 45–46
Pacerone. *See* Amiodarone
Pain management, 200–202
  acute pain and, 201
  biofeedback and, 201
  chest pain and, 242
  chronic pain and, 201
  deep breathing and, 202
  hypnosis and, 202
  meditation and, 202
  sleep and, 202
  surgery for, 202
  techniques for, 201–202
  topical agents for, 202
  types of pain and, 201
Part B, Medicare, 107
Part D, Medicare, 106–107
Partially hydrogenated oils, 221
Paying for care, 103–120
  assessing financial resources for, 104–105
  asset transfers and Medicaid eligibility in,
      113–114
  community-based services for, 118–119
  employment planning and, 114
  health maintenance organizations (HMOs) in,
      114–117
  hospice care and, 254–255
  housing options and, 62
  Medicaid for, 108–110, 112–114
  Medicare for, 105–108
  Older Americans Act and, 111
  public pay programs for, 105–111
  Social Security benefits for, 111–112
  Social Services Block Grant and, 111
  spousal impoverishment laws and, 109
  Veterans benefits for, 110–111
PCI. *See* percutaneous coronary intervention

Percutaneous coronary intervention (PCI), 45
Personal assistance programs, state and
    county, 94
Personal assistants, 97–100
  health care professionals as, 98–99
  interviewing, 97
  questions to ask before hiring, 100
  screening, 99–100
  tax rules concerning, 99
  where to find, 97–98
Personal hygiene, 164–170
Pharmacist, 80–81, 266
Physical examination, 27
Physical therapist, 72, 186–187, 266
Physical therapy, 186–189
  physical therapist's role in, 186–187
  range-of-motion (ROM) exercises in,
      187–189, 188!
Plan of care, 131–140
  emergency information form for, 139
  emergency preparedness in, 138
  information included in, 132–133
  medication management in, 135–138
  recording information in, 133–134
  sample of self-care log in, 134
Podiatrist, 266
Point of service (POS) plans, 115
Pool exercises, 232
Potassium, 43
Poultry, 224
Power of attorney, 123
Preparing for a doctor's visit, 74–75
Prescription drugs, Medicare Part D plan for,
    106–107
Pressure sores, 177–180, 180!
  common spots for, 180!
  prevention of, 178–179
  treatment of, 179–180
Primary care physician, 71
Prinivil. *See* lisinopril
Procainimide (Procanbid, Pronestyl), 42
Progression of heart failure, 4
Pronestyl. *See* Procainimide
Propafenone (Rythmol), 42
Protein, 213–214, 217
Psychiatrist, 266

mechanical heart pump in, 46
pacemakers in, 45–46
percutaneous coronary intervention (PCI)
        in, 45
stenting in, 45
valve surgery in, 45
ventricular assist device (VAD) in, 44
ventricular reconstrion (Dor procedure) in, 45
Swollen legs and feet, 170
Symptoms of heart failure, 4, 32–34
Systolic heart failure, 8
Systolic number in blood pressure, 10–11

Tambocor. *See* Flecainide
Taxes, in hiring a personal attendant, 99
Teeth. *See* oral/dental care
Telmisartan (Micardis), 41
Tests for heart failure, 27–29
Therapeutic diets, 215
Therapies, 185–191. *See also* physical therapy;
        occupational therapy
Thyroid disorders and heart failure, 12, 27
Toileting, 171–176
    bathroom toilet use in, 173
    bowel function, constipation, and, 175
    commode use in, 172
    diuretics and, 173
    hemorrhoids and, 175–176
    incontinence and, 173–174
    safety tips in, 172
    urinal use in, 171–172
    urinary tract infections and, 174
Topical pain medications, 202
Toprol. *See* Metoprolol
Torsemide (Demadex), 42
Training for caregiving duties, 100
Trandolapril (Mavik), 40
Trans fats, 221
Transportation services, 118, 206
Traveling, 206–207
Treatment of heart failure, 37–47
    cardiac health improvement and rehabilitation
            program (CHIRP) in, 47
    compliance with, 44
    diet in, 38–39

exercise in, 39
lifestyle changes in, 38–39
medications in, 38, 39–43
surgical options in, 44–46
Tricuspid valve, 7
Trust funds, 113
Tub baths, 166
Tuition help for continuing education, 198
Types of heart failure, 8–9

Uncontrollable risk factors, 18–19
Unsaturated fats, 220
Urinal use, 171–172
Urinary tract infections, 174
Urologist, 266

VAD. *See* ventricular assist device
Valsartan (Diovan), 41
Values history documents, 124
valves of the heart, 7–8, 12, 45
Vasotec. *See* Enalapril
Ventricle of heart, 7
Ventricular assist device (VAD), 44, 72
Ventricular reconstrion (Dor procedure), 45
Veterans benefits, 110–111
Viral illness and heart failure, 12
Vision care, 83–84

Warfarin. *See* Coumadin
Water pills. *See* diuretics
Water therapy/exercise, 232
Weight gain, 226. *See also* nutrition and diet
Weight loss, 219. *See also* nutrition and diet
Whole grains, 223
Wills, 123
Working with heart failure, 199–200. *See also*
        employment planning

X-rays, 28

Zaroxolyn. *See* Metolazone
Zebeta. *See* bisoprolol
Zestril. *See* lisinopril

Notes